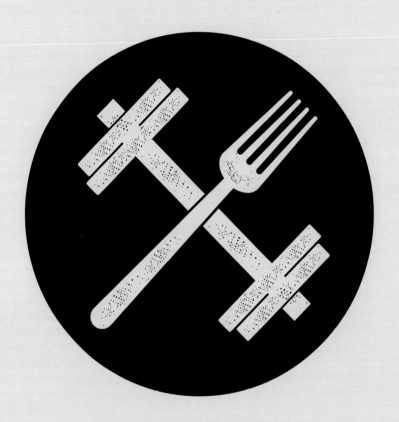

CLEAN SIMPLE EATS

WELCOME TO THE CSE SQUAD!

Hi! We're JJ and Erika, the husband and wife behind Clean Simple Eats! We are passionate about helping others elevate their lives through food and fitness, and we are here to prove that clean eating can be simple, fun and satisfying. That's why we've put a healthy spin on delicious comfort food recipes we all know and love (hello Boss Baked Mac & Cheese and Chocolate Waffles).

Frustrated by bland and boring diets, we started experimenting with recipes, substituting more healthful ingredients and before we knew it, Clean Simple Eats was born! But we couldn't stop there; we created four seasonal 7-week macro-balanced Meal Plans filled with hundreds of delicious, family-friendly recipes with just the right amount of protein, fat and carbs to keep your body fueled and satisfied. Our Meal Plans have proven to please even the pickiest of eaters (aka our four kiddos), and we guarantee that these meals will teach lifelong healthy habits.

Aside from our recipes, we've also created our own line of clean and tasty protein powders, supplements, and mixed nut butters (aka Off-Beat Butters, so yummy you'll want to eat them #bythespoonful). Our goal was (and is still) to create the best-tasting, highest quality products on the market, and we believe we did just that! Each small-batch flavor combo is unique, crave-worthy, and sure to leave you asking for more!

We believe that healthy habits + consistency over time yield the very best results, which means a sustainable diet is key. We also believe in the importance of a community that supports you. Here at CSE, we have a strong community called the CSE Squad! Our #CSESquad are strong and loyal rock stars who are willing to embrace a challenge—the #CSEChallenge.

It's been a great adventure, but the very best part is watching others take control of their narrative, reach goals, find inner confidence and transform their lives. That is the reason why we do what we do! We can't wait to be a part of your health and fitness journey!

Eat **clean,** keep it **simple**, get **results**.

In this plan, you'll find:

• 7 weeks of macro-friendly recipes that your whole family will love
• Menu planners and shopping lists for each week
• Weekly meal prep suggestions
• A Fast Food Macro Guide
• A Food Swaps List
• Calorie and macronutrient breakdowns for each individual recipe
• Calorie Quick List: determine how many meals/snacks you need
• Intro to Macros: how to customize this plan to fit your goals
• 11 workouts programmed by certified personal trainer, JJ Peterson

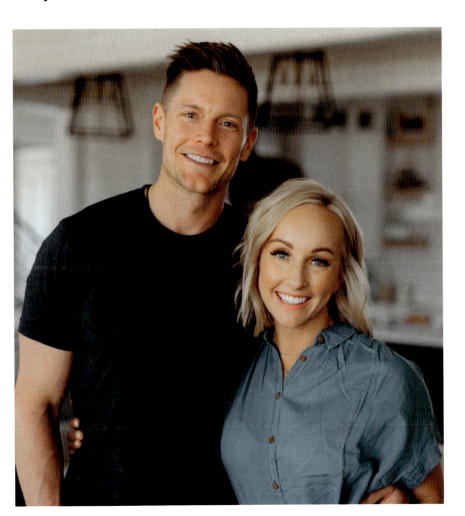

HOW TO USE THIS PLAN

• We designed this plan to make your weekly menu planning, grocery shopping and meal prep simple! Each grocery list includes enough groceries for breakfast, lunch and dinner for two adults each week. Make sure to add the ingredients for the snacks you choose each week to your shopping list! Snacks are not included on the grocery lists. You'll notice a menu pattern in this meal plan. Simple breakfasts on the weekdays, fun breakfasts on the weekends. Fresh, new dinners each night making enough to enjoy that dinner again for lunch the following day. Simple meal prep! Lunch is always ready to go! We built in two meals a week for dining out using our Fast Food Macros Guide.

• We encourage you to start at the beginning of the plan. Even if you're jumping into the challenge at a later date, start with Week 1. The groceries on each weekly grocery list will give you all the ingredients needed for meals that week through to Monday's lunch of the following week.

• The majority of the entrees in this meal plan make four servings. Breakfasts make anywhere from one to four servings. This meal plan was created to feed two adults. If you are feeding a family, you will want to double or triple each recipe to give you enough servings to feed each person. If you're using this plan by yourself, you can either cut each recipe and grocery list in half or keep the portions where they're at and cook fewer meals each week. Before making adjustments, make sure to check how many servings each meal makes and how many caloires you need per day to reach your goal.

• One note about the "dine out" meals. We wouldn't recommend eating more than your maintenance calories for the day, especially if your goal is weight loss. For example, if your maintenance calories equal 2,000, you would want to stick to 2,000 calories or less for the day (including your dine out meal) to keep you on track to reaching your goals. You wouldn't want to ruin all the progress you've made for the week all in one meal! It can happen fast! Refer to the "Tips for Dining Out"page and our "Fast Food Macros Guide" included in this book to help you stay mindful when dining out.

• If there are meals you don't prefer, remember that all meals are interchangeable. You can swap out any meal you'd like for another. You can always visit our website, cleansimpleeats.com/resources to download your own blank menu planner and grocery list. Our CSE+ App also makes menu planning super easy!

• Make sure to familiarize yourself with the Food Prep Guide at the beginning of this book. There are weekly meal prep recommendations found in this section that, if followed, will save you a ton of time and help to keep you on point during the challenge.

• The HIIT workouts that you'll find toward the back of the book are completely optional, but we know you'll love them! These workouts were programmed by JJ (who is a certified personal trainer) and have been designed to burn fat and build muscle. Plan to repeat the Monday workout for 7 Mondays in a row, the Tuesday workout for 7 Tuesdays, etc. Track your progress and improvements each week.

LET'S GET STARTED!

1. Grab a buddy to start this plan with you. Having an accountability partner will double your chances of success!

2. Before you shop, read over the provided weekly shopping list and cross out any items that you might already have on hand (we suggest you do this every week before shopping). Clean out your pantry and fridge. Throw away any junk food or trigger foods that might derail your progress during the next 7 weeks.

3. Drink lots of water. We suggest that you drink half of your bodyweight in ounces of water everyday. Even more if you are active!

4. Take before pictures and measurements. Pictures and measurements are the best way to show how far you have come.

WE BELIEVE IN YOU! YOU'VE GOT THIS!

A BIT ABOUT MACROS

This is a "macro-based" meal plan, meaning every recipe has a balanced macronutrient ratio of 40% carbs, 30% protein and 30% fat. This 40/30/30 approach has been proven time and time again to offer balance and lifelong sustainability. The most beautiful part about the CSE meal plans (minus the food itself) is the fact that you can eat like this forever! This meal plan was designed to help you AND your family gain lasting healthy habits in the kitchen and a positive relationship with food. Don't worry too much about the science behind this meal plan. We've done all the hard work for you!

What are macros and why do they need to be balanced? Macronutrients are nutrients that provide calories or energy. Nutrients are substances needed for growth, metabolism, and for other body functions. Since "macro" means large, macronutrients are nutrients needed in large amounts.

There are three macronutrients:

- **Protein**
- **Fat**
- **Carbohydrates**

While each of these macros provide calories, the amount of calories that each one provides varies.

Carbohydrates: 4 calories per gram
Protein: 4 calories per gram
Fat: 9 calories per gram

This means that if you looked at the Nutrition Facts label of a product and it said 12 grams of carbs, 0 grams of fat, and 0 grams of protein per serving, you would know that this food has about 48 calories per serving (12 grams carbs multiplied by 4 calories for each gram of carbohydrate = 48 calories).

WHY DO WE NEED CARBOHYDRATES?
• The body's preferred source of fuel and energy
• Can be easily used by the body for energy
• All of the tissues and cells in our body can use glucose for energy
• Needed for the central nervous system, the kidneys, the brain, and the muscles (including the heart) to function properly.
• Can be stored in the muscles and liver for later use of energy
• Important in intestinal health and waste elimination

Carbohydrates are mainly found in starchy foods (like grains and potatoes), fruits, milk, and yogurt. Other foods like vegetables, beans, nuts, seeds, and cottage cheese contain carbohydrates, but in lesser amounts.

WHY DO WE NEED PROTEIN?
• Tissue repair
• Immune function
• Making essential hormones and enzymes
• Building and preserving lean muscle mass
• Growth (especially for children, teens, and pregnant women)

Protein is found in meats, poultry, fish, tofu, cheese, milk, nuts, legumes, and in smaller quantities in starchy foods and vegetables.

WHY DO WE NEED FAT?
• Normal growth, development and cell function
• Energy (fat is the most concentrated source of energy)
• Absorbing certain vitamins (like vitamins A, D, E, K, and carotenoids)
• Maintaining cell membranes for healthy skin and other tissues
• Needed for proper functioning of nerves and brain
• Regulate hormones and many bodily processes
• Providing taste, consistency, and stability to foods

Fat is found in meat, poultry, nuts, milk products, butters, oils, fish, grain products and salad dressings. There are three main types of fat: trans fat, saturated fat, and unsaturated fat. Completely eliminate trans fats from your diet if possible. These fats are found in fried foods, processed foods, fast foods, and snack foods. Limit the saturated fats coming from animal products and go with coconut oil! Stick to good, healthy fats that you find in avocados, avocado oil, EVOO, nuts, and nut butters.

CUSTOMIZE YOUR PLAN

DOWNLOAD THE CSE+ APP

Available in the App Store or Google Play. Input your personal information to customize your goals and you're all set! For more information, visit cleansimpleeats.com/pages/app

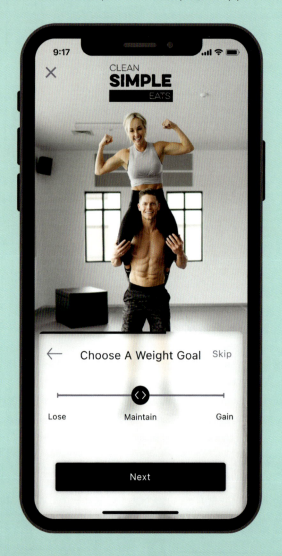

MACRO QUICK LIST

CHOOSE ONE OF THE TWO OPTIONS LISTED BELOW YOUR CUSTOM
CALORIE COUNT TO REACH YOUR DAILY MACRO GOAL

 1250 - 1300 CALORIES: 42F / 125C / 94P
3 MEAL SERVINGS + 1 SNACK SERVING
3 MEAL SERVINGS + 2 POWER BITES

 1500 - 1550 CALORIES: 50F / 150C / 113P
3 MEAL SERVINGS + 2 SNACK SERVINGS
3 MEAL SERVINGS + 1 SNACK SERVING + 2 POWER BITES

 1750 - 1800 CALORIES: 58F / 175C / 131P
3 MEAL SERVINGS + 3 SNACK SERVINGS
3 MEAL SERVINGS + 2 SNACK SERVINGS + 2 POWER BITES

 2000 - 2050 CALORIES: 67F / 200C / 150P
3 MEAL SERVINGS + 3 SNACK SERVINGS + 2 POWER BITES
4 MEAL SERVINGS + 2 SNACK SERVINGS + 1 POWER BITE

 2250 - 2300 CALORIES: 75F / 225C / 169P
4 MEAL SERVINGS + 3 SNACK SERVINGS + 1 POWER BITE
3 MEAL SERVINGS + 4 SNACK SERVINGS + 2 POWER BITES

 2500 - 2550 CALORIES: 83F / 250C / 188P
5 MEAL SERVINGS + 2 SNACK SERVINGS + 2 POWER BITES
6 MEAL SERVINGS + 1 SNACK SERVING + 1 POWER BITE

 2750 - 2800 CALORIES: 92F / 275C / 206P
6 MEAL SERVINGS + 2 SNACK SERVINGS + 2 POWER BITES
6 MEAL SERVINGS + 3 SNACK SERVINGS

 3000 - 3050 CALORIES: 100F / 300C / 225P
6 MEAL SERVINGS + 4 SNACK SERVINGS
6 MEAL SERVINGS + 3 SNACK SERVINGS + 2 POWER BITES

The ideas, concepts and opinions expressed in all Clean Simple Eats meal plans, books and other media are intended to be used for educational purposes only. The books and meal plans are sold with the understanding that authors and publisher are not rendering medical advice of any kind, nor are the books or meal plans intended to replace medical advice, nor to diagnose, prescribe or treat any disease, condition, illness or injury. By my use of any of the products and/or programs of Clean Simple Eats, I am agreeing to assume all of the risks associated with such use. I further agree to waive, release, and discharge Clean Simple Eats from any and all liability arising from its negligence or fault.

It is imperative that before beginning any diet or exercise program, including any aspect of the Clean Simple Eats program, you receive full medical clearance from a licensed physician.

Authors and publisher claim no responsibility to any person or entity for any liability, loss or damage caused or alleged to be caused directly or indirectly as a result of the use, application or interpretation of the material in the books or meal plan.

The Food and Drug Administration has not evaluated the statements contained in any Clean Simple Eats books, meal plans, or other media.

This book, and any other Clean Simple Eats seasonal meal plan or book, is protected under copyright laws and may not be duplicated, shared, copied or plagiarized, under any circumstance, in digital or bound form.

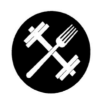

RECIPE
INDEX

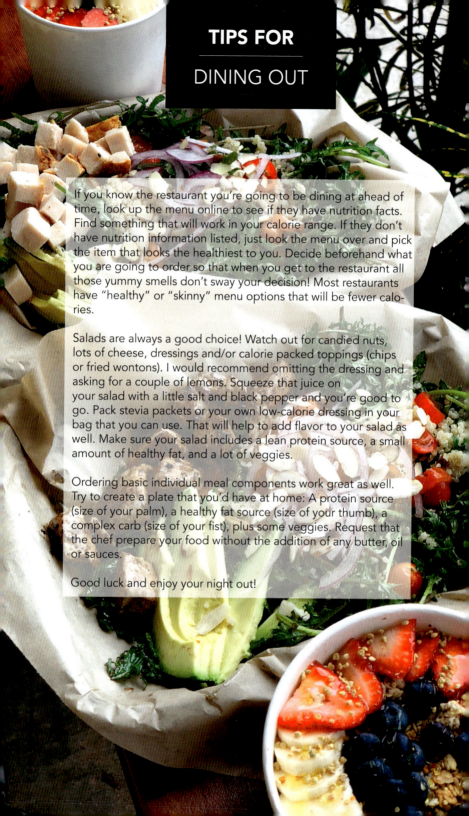

TIPS FOR

DINING OUT

If you know the restaurant you're going to be dining at ahead of time, look up the menu online to see if they have nutrition facts. Find something that will work in your calorie range. If they don't have nutrition information listed, just look the menu over and pick the item that looks the healthiest to you. Decide beforehand what you are going to order so that when you get to the restaurant all those yummy smells don't sway your decision! Most restaurants have "healthy" or "skinny" menu options that will be fewer calories.

Salads are always a good choice! Watch out for candied nuts, lots of cheese, dressings and/or calorie packed toppings (chips or fried wontons). I would recommend omitting the dressing and asking for a couple of lemons. Squeeze that juice on your salad with a little salt and black pepper and you're good to go. Pack stevia packets or your own low-calorie dressing in your bag that you can use. That will help to add flavor to your salad as well. Make sure your salad includes a lean protein source, a small amount of healthy fat, and a lot of veggies.

Ordering basic individual meal components work great as well. Try to create a plate that you'd have at home: A protein source (size of your palm), a healthy fat source (size of your thumb), a complex carb (size of your fist), plus some veggies. Request that the chef prepare your food without the addition of any butter, oil or sauces.

Good luck and enjoy your night out!

FAST FOOD
MACRO GUIDE

Café Rio
• Grilled Chicken Salad, no tortilla, rice, lettuce, pico, cilantro, lime, bring 2 T. Bolthouse Farms Cilantro Avocado Dressing
352 calories | 15F | 33C | 22P
• Grilled Chicken Tostada on white corn tortilla, rice, lettuce, pico, cilantro, lime
408 calories | 14F | 37C | 37P
• Grilled Chicken Tacos (2) on white corn tortilla, rice, lettuce, pico, cilantro, lime
466 calories | 10F | 40C | 58P
• Grilled Salmon Tacos (2) on white corn tortillas, rice, lettuce, pico, cilantro, lime
352 calories | 10F | 36C | 34P
• Grilled Steak Tacos (2) on white corn tortillas, rice, lettuce, pico, cilantro, lime
378 calories | 12F | 34C | 36P
• Mahi Mahi Tacos (2) on white corn tortillas, rice, lettuce, pico, cilantro, lime
278 calories | 6F | 30C | 30P

Café Zupas
• Asian Citrus Chicken Salad – large, no dressing *270 calories | 13F | 19C | 20P*
• BBQ Chicken Salad – large, no dressing
310 calories | 10F | 34C | 18P
• Strawberry Harvest Chicken – large, no dressing *260 calories | 12F | 19C | 18P*
• Chocolate Covered Strawberry
45 calories | 2F | 7C | 1P

California Pizza Kitchen
• Sesame Dumplings
328 calories | 8F | 45C | 19P
• OG BBQ Chicken Pizza - 2 Slices
378 calories | 10F | 50C | 22P
• Cali Veggie Pizza - 2 Slices
386 calories | 10F | 50C | 24P
• Jamaican Jerk Pizza - 2 Slices
430 calories | 14F | 52C | 24P
• Wild Mushroom Pizza
+ Chicken - 2 Slices
397 calories | 13F | 46C | 24P

Cheesecake Factory
• Skinnylicious Mexican Chicken Lettuce Wraps
220 calories | 9F | 14C | 24P
• Skinnylicious Turkey Burger
336 calories | 8F | 38C | 28P

Chick-Fil-A
• Grilled Chicken Sandwich, no sauce
320 calories | 5F | 40aC | 30P
• Asian Salad, no dressing
330 calories | 13F | 24C | 29P
• Grilled Chicken Cool Wrap
330 calories | 12F | 28C | 38P
• Chicken Tortilla Soup, medium
260 calories | 6F | 29C | 22P

Chipotle
• Chicken Salad: lettuce, chicken, ½ brown rice, ½ black beans, tomato salsa
360 calories | 10F | 30C | 38P

Corelife Eatery
• Big Spicy Chicken & Ancient Grains Bowl
290 calories | 8F | 29C | 26P
• Big Spicy Thai Chicken & Rice Noodles Bowl
310 calories | 4F | 47C | 23P
• Small Poke Bowl
350 calories | 22F | 21C | 28P
• Big Berry Quinoa Chicken Bowl
420 calories | 17F | 41C | 29P
• Small BBQ Ranch Chicken Bowl
430 calories | 10F | 56C | 29P
• Small Spicy Chicken Bowl
360 calories | 11F | 40C | 26P
• Big Chicken & Rice Noodle Broth Bowl
310 calories | 1.5F | 40C | 31P
• Small Chicken Tortilla & Chipotle Broth Bowl
300 calories | 5F | 30C | 31P
• Small Spicy Ginger & Steak Rice Noodle Broth Bowl
320 calories | 11F | 24C | 32P

Costa Vida

• Taco, one: Black beans, chicken or mahi mahi, lettuce, lime, pico de gallo w/corn tortilla: *320 calories | 6F | 44C | 23P*
w/whole wheat tortilla:
350 calories | 10F | 42C | 24P
• Raspberry Chicken Salad, Small:
Whole wheat tortilla, chicken, black beans, lettuce, raspberry chipotle sauce, pico
380 calories | 10F | 51C | 23P
• Baja Bowl: Rice, chicken, tomatillo cilantro sauce, lettuce, pico de gallo
380 calories | 10F | 38C | 33P

Culver's

• Grilled Chicken Sandwich
387 calories | 7F | 40C | 41P
• Beef Pot Roast Sandwich
410 calories | 13F | 40C | 31P
• Grilled Chicken Caesar Salad
308 calories | 12F | 17C | 33P
• Garden Fresco & Grilled Chicken Salad
350 calories | 14F | 15C | 44P

The Habit Burger Grill

• Lettuce Wrap Charburger
352 calories | 19F | 3C | 18P
• Chargrilled Ahi Tuna Sandwich
390 calories | 10F | 51C | 28P
• Grilled Chicken Salad, no dressing
410 calories | 15F | 35C | 35P

Einstein Bros. Bagels

• Thintastic Turkey Sausage & Cheddar Egg White Sandwich
330 calories | 10F | 35C | 25P
• Thintastic Southwest Egg White Sandwich
330 calories | 10F | 35C | 24P
• Thintastic Santa Fe Egg White Sandwich
410 calories | 16F | 42C | 25P
• Thintastic Tasty Turkey Sandwich
431 calories | 15F | 45C | 29P
• Thintastic Buffalo Chicken Sandwich
430 calories | 12F | 50C | 32P

Fueled Fresh Kitchen

• Breakfast Hash
404 calories | 8F | 36C | 43P

• Breakfast Sandwich w/sausage
362 calories | 12F | 33C | 30P
• Greek Yogurt
360 calories | 7F | 49C | 29P
• Fueled Veggie Omelet
286 calories | 7F | 31C | 25P
• PB Vacation Shake
409 calories | 9F | 41C | 46P
• Chocolate PB Love Shake
419 calories | 9F | 44C | 46P
• Island Breeze Shake
400 calories | 12F | 47C | 32P
• Fueled Beast Shake
312 calories | 16F | 19C | 30P
• Yoda Shake
328 calories | 15F | 26C | 30P
• Very Berry Acai Smoothie
309 calories | 9F | 30C | 28P
• Tropical Paradise Acai Smoothie
363 calories | 13F | 35C | 28P
• Nuts N' Berries Acai Smoothie
436 calories | 15F | 32C | 45P
• Blackened BBQ Chicken Bowl
*without carb option
321 calories | 4F | 29C | 43P
• Chicken Curry Bowl
*without carb option
325 calories | 9F | 17C | 44P
• Skinny Salmon Bowl
386 calories | 19F | 17C | 39P
• Teriyaki Bowl
*without carb option
312 calories | 5F | 22C | 43P
• Poke Tacos
376 calories | 12F | 43C | 28P
• Bruschetta Steak Tacos
371 calories | 14F | 38C | 27P

In 'N' Out

• Double Hamburger protein style, add mustard instead of spread
340 calories | 23F | 11C | 33P
• Hamburger w/mustard & ketchup instead of spread
310 calories | 10F | 41C | 16P

Jack's
• Grilled Chicken Salad
310 calories | 13F | 18C | 34P
• Grilled Chicken Sandwich
410 calories | 17F | 35C | 29P

Kneaders
• ½ Turkey, Bacon, Avocado Sandwich
370 calories | 15F | 42C | 21P
• Turkey Cranberry Sunflower Salad, no dressing
340 calories | 15F | 26C | 26P
• White Bean Chicken Chili
190 calories | 3F | 19C | 21P

McDonald's
• Egg White Delight McMuffin
250 calories | 7F | 30C | 18P
• Fruit & Maple Oatmeal, no brown sugar, Add ½ serving
CSE protein powder
320 calories | 4F | 51C | 17P
• Southwest Salad w/ grilled chicken, no dressing
290 calories | 8F | 28C | 27P
• Bacon Ranch Salad with Grilled Chicken, no dressing
230 calories | 9F | 10C | 30P
• Honey Mustard Snack Wrap, Grilled or Chipotle BBQ Snack Wrap, Grilled
250 calories | 8F | 27C | 16P
• Grilled Chicken Sandwich, no sauce
350 calories | 9F | 42C | 28P
• McWrap Sweet Chili Chicken
360 calories | 9F | 43C | 26P

MOD Pizza
• Mini Jasper
340 calories | 11F | 41C | 18P
• Mini Dillon James, add chicken
410 calories | 12.5F | 51C | 21.5P
• Mini Caspian
420 calories | 13F | 54C | 22P
• Mini Chicken, Mushroom & Tomato
375 calories | 11F | 50C | 20P
• Mini Calexico
370 calories | 13F | 41C | 22P

• Mini Maddy, add chicken
380 calories | 10F | 40C | 30P

Panda Express
• Grilled Teriyaki Chicken 6oz
+ Mixed Veggies
378 calories | 13.5F | 24C | 40P
• Grilled Asian Chicken 6oz
+ Mixed Veggies
378 calories | 13.5F | 24C | 40P
• String Bean Chicken 5.6oz
+ Mixed Veggies
274 calories | 9.5F | 29C | 18P

PDQ
• Classic Salad, Grilled Chicken
270 calories | 11F | 11C | 34P
• Grilled Chicken Tenders, 3ct.
180 calories | 2F | 12C | 31P
• Cali Club Sandwich, Lettuce Wrap
300 calories | 13F | 17C | 33P
• Grilled Cali Bowl, No Rice
430 calories | 15F | 40C | 37P
• Grilled Chicken Sandwich, Brioche Bun w/Honey Mustard
400 calories | 13F | 39C | 31P

Pei Wei
(omit rice and noodles in all entrees)
• Small Sesame Chicken salad or lettuce wrapped:
410 *calories | 13F | 44C | 26P*
• Small Sweet n' Sour Chicken salad or lettuce wrapped:
290 calories | 3F | 42C | 24P
• Small Mongolian Chicken salad or lettuce wrapped:
330 calories | 13F | 30C | 23P
• Small Thai Dynamite Chicken salad or lettuce wrapped:
280 calories | 8F | 25C | 26P
• Regular Lemon Pepper Chicken salad or lettuce wrapped:
400 calories | 4.5F | 44C | 43P

Panera Bread
- Mediterranean Scrambled Egg White Wrap
270 calories | 8F | 33C | 20P
- Greek Yogurt w/Mixed Berries
300 calories | 10F | 39C | 14P
- Mediterranean Scrambled Strawberry Poppyseed Salad
210 calories | 11F | 28C | 20P
- Seasonal Greens Salad w/Chicken
255 calories | 12F | 20C | 20.5P
- Lentil Quinoa Broth Bowl w/Chicken
380 calories | 8F | 45C | 32P
- Soba Noodle Broth Bowl w/Chicken
360 calories | 9F | 43C | 28P

Pizzeria Limone
- Caesar Salad, Full + chicken w/ 2 oz. Lemon Vinaigrette Dressing
400 calories | 18F | 37C | 23P
- Tre Sorelle Salad, half + chicken w/ 2 oz. Lemon Vinaigrette Dressing
395 calories | 18F | 37C | 21P
- Viola Pizza - ½ pizza
410 calories | 16F | 48C | 18P
- Verdure Pizza - ½ pizza
395 calories | 15F | 50C | 15P

Potbelly Sandwich Shop
- Farmhouse Salad
321 calories | 15F | 11C | 35P
- Skinny T-K-Y
294 calories | 6F | 40C | 22P
- Buffalo Grilled Chicken Sandwich on multigrain wheat
332 calories | 11F | 39C | 21P
- Skinny Beef Sandwich on multigrain ThinCut wheat
340 calories | 10F | 39C | 22P
- Turkey Breast Sandwich on multigrain wheat
442 calories | 11F | 58C | 36P

Protein Foundry
- Lush Shake Out, 16 oz.
325 calories | 8F | 37C | 29P
- Raspberry Cheesecake Shake Out, 16 oz.
330 calories | 8F | 36C | 30P
- Super M(atcha) Shake Out, 16 oz.
340 calories | 5F | 49C | 29P
- Aphrodite Bowl, vanilla
325 calories | 8F | 52C | 17P
- Athena Bowl, vanilla
360 calories | 11F | 52C | 18P

Protein House
- SHRDD Veggie Omelette w/side fruit
261 calories | 7F | 32C | 23P
- Super Bird Omelette w/side fruit
307 calories | 7F | 23C | 39P
- Hulk Protein Shake
430 calories | 11F | 56C | 31P
- Apple Butter Shake
463 calories | 12F | 54C | 31P
- Vanilla Gorilla Frap
313 calories | 10F | 28C | 26P
- Mocha Loca Frap
310 calories | 10F | 27C | 29P
- Aloha Burger (whole wheat bun)
401 calories | 7F | 42C | 46P
- Portobello Sandwich
264 calories | 5F | 13C | 44P

Shake Shack
- Burger Patty on gluten-free bun, no cheese, add ketchup and veggies of choice
360 calories | 15.5F | 32C | 21P
- Burger Patty on lettuce wrap, no cheese, add ketchup and veggies of choice
196 calories | 12F | 2C | 20P
- Chicken Bites
300 calories | 15F | 18C | 22P
- Chicken Dog
310 calories | 13F | 27C | 24P
- Chicken Shack-Cago Dog
330 calories | 13F | 31C | 24P

Starbucks

- Blueberry Muesli & Yogurt Bowl
310 calories | 1.5F | 57C | 17P
- Blueberries & Honey Greek Yogurt Parfait
240 calories | 2.5F | 42C | 14P
- Lemon Crunch Yogurt Parfait
340 calories | 13F | 38C | 18P
- Berry Trio Parfait
240 calories | 2.5F | 39C | 14P
- Mango & Coconut Yogurt Bowl
290 calories | 6F | 57C | 12P
- Classic Oatmeal + 1 serving CSE Protein
270 calories | 2.5F | 37C | 25P
- Hearty Blueberry Oatmeal + 1 serving CSE Simply Vanilla Protein
330 calories | 2.5F | 52C | 25P
- Bacon Gouda & Egg Sandwich
370 calories | 19F | 32C | 18P
- Spinach Feta & Egg White Wrap
290 calories | 10F | 33C | 19P
- Ham & Cheese Croissant
320 calories | 17F | 28C | 14P
- Turkey Bacon & Egg White Breakfast Sandwich
220 calories | 5F | 26C | 18P
- Tomato & Mozzarella Sandwich
350 calories | 13F | 42C | 15P
- Honey BBQ Sriracha Chicken Sandwich
370 calories | 8F | 54C | 22P
- Chicken & Quinoa Protein Bowl
420 calories | 17F | 42C | 27P
- Za'atar Chicken & Lemon Tahini Salad
430 calories | 21F | 42C | 21P
- Seasoned Turkey & Green Pepper Pico Salad
390 calories | 18F | 30C | 28P
- Cage-Free Eggs & Seasoned Grains Side Salad
360 calories | 18F | 33C | 17P

Subway

- 3" Egg White Sandwich, double egg whites, Artisan Flatbread, cheddar cheese, avocado
244 calories | 8F | 23C | 20P
- 6" Oven Roasted Chicken Breast Sandwich, honey wheat bread, provolone cheese, veggies, mustard, salt & pepper
320 calories | 7F | 40C | 27P
- 6" Sweet Onion Chicken Teriyaki Sandwich, honey wheat bread, swiss cheese, veggies, sweet onion sauce, salt & pepper
360 calories | 8F | 48C | 29P
- 6" Roast Beef Sandwich honey wheat bread, pepper jack cheese, veggies, mustard, salt & pepper
340 calories | 9F | 40C | 29P
- 6" Rotisserie Chicken Sandwich, honey wheat bread, pepper jack cheese, veggies, mustard, salt & pepper
330 calories | 8F | 41C | 25P
- 6" Subway Club Sandwich, honey wheat bread, American cheese, veggies, mustard, salt & pepper
340 calories | 8F | 42C | 26P
- Rotisserie Style Chicken Salad, veggies, feta cheese, Subway Vinaigrette
310 calories | 16F | 14C | 28P

Wendy's

- Parmesan Caesar Chicken Salad (half size)
320 calories | 20F | 9C | 29P
- Apple Pecan Chicken Salad (half size)
340 calories | 17F | 29C | 20P
- Harvest Chicken Salad (half size)
330 calories | 15F | 25C | 22P
- Southwest Avocado Chicken Salad (half size)
310 calories | 21F | 10C | 22P
- Large Chili
250 calories | 6F | 29C | 21P
- Grilled Chicken Wrap
300 calories | 13F | 26C | 20P
- Grilled Chicken Sandwich
380 calories | 10F | 38C | 35P

WEEK 1

MENU PLANNER

	BREAKFAST	SNACK	LUNCH	SNACK	DINNER	*SNACK
MON	Raspberry Almond Oats P99	Choose from snack options	Buffalo Chicken & Pesto Sandwich P129	Choose from snack options	Pasta E Fagioli P131	*Choose from snack options
TUES	Raspberry Almond Oats	Choose from snack options	Pasta E Fagioli	Choose from snack options	Rotisserie Chicken Tacos P133	*Choose from snack options
WED	Raspberry Almond Oats	Choose from snack options	Rotisserie Chicken Tacos	Choose from snack options	BBQ Chicken Chopped Salad P135	*Choose from snack options
THURS	Raspberry Almond Oats	Choose from snack options	BBQ Chicken Chopped Salad	Choose from snack options	Aloha Chicken Kabobs P137	*Choose from snack options
FRI	Raspberry Almond Oats	Choose from snack options	Aloha Chicken Kabobs	Choose from snack options	DINE OUT	N/A
SAT	Breakfast Tacos P101	Choose from snack options	Buffalo Chicken & Pesto Sandwich	Choose from snack options	Cheesy Broccoli & Bacon Penne P139	*Choose from snack options
SUN	Breakfast Tacos	Choose from snack options	Cheesy Broccoli & Bacon Penne	Choose from snack options	Parmesan Chicken P141	*Choose from snack options

*Be sure this snack fits into your daily calorie allotment.

WEEK 1 GROCERY LIST | Serves 2 adults for the week

PRODUCE
Asparagus, 48 spears
Avocado, 2
Bell Pepper, Red, 1
Broccoli, 4 cups
Cabbage, Red, 1 cup
Carrots, 2 medium
Celery, 2 sticks
Cilantro, 1 bunch
Clementine Oranges, 8
Garlic, 3 cloves
Lemon, 1
Lettuce, Shredded, 2 cups
Limes, 2
Onion, Red, 1
Onions, Yellow, 2
Pineapple, 1
Potatoes, Baby Red, 18 oz. (~1 ¼ lb.)
Raspberries, Fresh or Frozen, 3 ⅓ cups
Spinach, 11 cups
Tomatoes, Vine, 4

MEAT & SEAFOOD
Beef, Lean, Ground, 12 oz. (¾ lb.)
Chicken Breast, 32 oz. (2 lbs.)
Chicken Tenderloins, 9 oz. (~ ½ lb.)
Rotisserie Chicken, 1
Turkey Bacon, 6 slices

REFRIGERATED
Almond Milk, Unsweetened, ¼ cup
Bolthouse Farms Cilantro Avocado
    Dressing, ½ cup
Cheese, Laughing Cow, Light, 8 wedges
Cheese, Mozzarella, Shredded, ¾ cup
Cheese, Parmesan, Grated, ¾ cup
Cheese, Pepper Jack, Slices, 4
Eggs, 19
Egg Whites, 10 (1 ¼ cups liquid)
Guacamole, ¼ cup
Greek Yogurt, Plain, Nonfat, 2 ⅔ cups
Pesto Sauce, 2 Tbs.
Pico De Gallo, ½ cup

PANTRY
Almonds, Sliced, 6 oz.
Balsamic Glaze, 4 tsp.
Beans, Black, 1 cup
Beans, Great Northern, ½ cup
Beans, Red Kidney, ½ cup
Cashews, ½ cup
Coconut Aminos or Soy Sauce, 1 Tbs.
Coconut Milk, Canned, Full Fat, 1 can
Coconut, Shredded, Unsweetened, 2 Tbs.
CSE Simply Vanilla Protein Powder, 5
    servings
Honey, Raw, ½ Tbs.
Hot Sauce, Frank's, 4 tsp.
Oats, Old-Fashioned Rolled, 3 ⅓ cups
OffBeat Salted Caramel Butter
    or Almond Butter, Natural, 5 Tbs.
OffBeat Sweet Classic Peanut Butter,
    Buckeye Brownie Peanut Butter, or
    Natural Peanut Butter, 4 Tbs.
Olive Oil, 3 Tbs.
Pasta, Macaroni or Ditalini, 2 oz.
Pasta, Whole Wheat, Penne, 4 oz.
Rice, White, Jasmine, 6 Tbs. uncooked
Salsa, 4 Tbs.
Stubb's Original BBQ Sauce, ½ cup
Tomato Sauce, 1 cup
Tomatoes, Diced, Canned, 2 cups
Tortillas, Corn, 16
Vegetable Broth, ½ cup
Vinegar, Rice, 1 tsp.
Vinegar, White Wine, 2 tsp.
Whole Wheat Hamburger Buns, 4 (140 cals)

SWEETENERS, SEASONINGS & SPICES
Almond Extract, 1 ¼ tsp.
Basil, Dried, 1 tsp.
Black Pepper
Garlic, Granulated, ¼ tsp.
Ginger, Ground, ½ tsp.
Oregano, Dried, ½ tsp.
Sea Salt
Stevia, Liquid Drops, Vanilla, optional
Taco Seasoning, 1-2 Tbs.
Thyme, Dried, ½ tsp.

FREEZER
Corn, Yellow, Sweet, 1 cup
Ezekiel Bread, 1 slice

MISC.
Cooking Spray
Parchment Paper
Skewer Sticks

Remember to purchase ingredients for your selected weekly snacks!

WEEK 2

MENU PLANNER

	BREAKFAST	SNACK	LUNCH	SNACK	DINNER	*SNACK
MON	Cinnamon Roll Shake P103	Choose from snack options	Parmesan Chicken P141	Choose from snack options	Balsamic Chicken Chopped Salad P143	*Choose from snack options
TUES	Cinnamon Roll Shake	Choose from snack options	Balsamic Chicken Chopped Salad	Choose from snack options	Citrus Salmon Tacos P145	*Choose from snack options
WED	Cinnamon Roll Shake	Choose from snack options	Citrus Salmon Tacos	Choose from snack options	Roasted Winter Squash & Sausage P147	*Choose from snack options
THURS	Cinnamon Roll Shake	Choose from snack options	Roasted Winter Squash & Sausage	Choose from snack options	Sweet Potato Pie P149	*Choose from snack options
FRI	Cinnamon Roll Shake	Choose from snack options	Sweet Potato Pie	Choose from snack options	DINE OUT	N/A
SAT	Chocolate Waffles P105	Choose from snack options	FAST FOOD MACRO GUIDE	Choose from snack options	Mexican Fajita Bowl P151	*Choose from snack options
SUN	Chocolate Waffles	Choose from snack options	Mexican Fajita Bowl	Choose from snack options	Pesto Tomato & Broccoli Fusilli P153	*Choose from snack options

***Be sure this snack fits into your daily calorie allotment.**

20

PRODUCE
Avocado, 2
Bananas, 5
Bell Pepper, Red, 1
Broccoli, 4 cups
Brussels Sprouts, 4 cups
Butternut Squash, 1 ½ lbs.
Cabbage, 2 cups
Carrots, 5 oz.
Cilantro, 1 bunch
Garlic, 4 cloves
Green Onions, 1 bunch
Limes, 3
Onion, Red, 2
Onion, Yellow, 1
Rosemary, 1 bunch (or 1 tsp. dried)
Sage, 1 bunch (or 1 tsp. dried)
Spring Salad Mix, 8 cups
Sweet Potatoes, 2 ¼ lb.
Tomatoes, Cherry, 1 cup
Tomatoes, Vine, 2

MEAT & SEAFOOD
Chicken Breast, 32 oz. (2 lbs.)
Chicken Sausage, Large (160 cals each)
   (Aidells, Coleman, Simple Truth), 5
   links
Salmon, Wild Caught, 12 oz (¾ lb.)
Turkey Bacon, 8 slices

REFRIGERATED
Almond Milk, Unsweetened, 7 ½ cups
Cheese, Feta, ¼ cup
Cheese, Mozzarella, Shredded, ½ cup
Cheese, Parmesan, Grated, ¾ cup
Eggs, 6
Greek Yogurt, Plain, Nonfat, 3 cups
Guacamole, 1 cup
Pesto Sauce, 4 Tbs.
Spray Whipped Cream, 8 Tbs.

PANTRY
Beans, Black, 1 cup
Cocoa Powder, 2 Tbs.

Coconut Sugar, 10 tsp.
CSE Brownie Batter Protein, 1 serving
CSE Simply Vanilla Protein Powder,
   7 ½ servings
CSE Vanilla Pancake & Waffle Mix, 1 ¾ cups
Honey, Raw, 2 tsp.
Oats, Old-Fashioned Rolled, 1 ½ cups
OffBeat Cinnamon Bun Butter, 10 Tbs.
   or Neufchâtel Cream Cheese, 30 Tbs.
OffBeat Sweet Classic Peanut Butter
   or Peanut Butter, Natural, ¼ cup
Olive Oil, 2 Tbs.
Pasta, Fusilli, Whole Grain, 5 oz. uncooked
Rice, White, Jasmine, ⅓ cup uncooked
Salsa, ½ cup
Stubb's Citrus & Onion Sauce, ½ cup
Tortillas, Corn, 8
Vinegar, Balsamic, ¼ cup
Zero Calorie Syrup of Choice

SWEETENERS, SEASONINGS & SPICES
Black Pepper
Cinnamon, Ground, 10 tsp.
Cumin, Ground, dash
Italian Seasoning, 1 tsp.
Red Pepper Flakes, optional
Sea Salt
Stevia in the Raw, to taste
Stevia, Liquid Drops, Vanilla, optional
Taco Seasoning, 1 Tbs.

MISC.
Cooking Spray
Parchment Paper
Ziploc Bags, Large

Remember to purchase ingredients for your selected weekly snacks!

WEEK 3

MENU PLANNER

	BREAKFAST	SNACK	LUNCH	SNACK	DINNER	*SNACK
MON	Gingerbread Cookie Oatmeal P107	Choose from snack options	Pesto Tomato & Broccoli Fusilli P153	Choose from snack options	Chicken Stir-Fry P155	*Choose from snack options
TUES	Gingerbread Cookie Oatmeal	Choose from snack options	Chicken Stir-Fry	Choose from snack options	Taco Salad P157	*Choose from snack options
WED	Gingerbread Cookie Oatmeal	Choose from snack options	Taco Salad	Choose from snack options	Salmon & Greens Spaghetti P159	*Choose from snack options
THURS	Gingerbread Cookie Oatmeal	Choose from snack options	Salmon & Greens Spaghetti	Choose from snack options	Chicken Pad Thai P161	*Choose from snack options
FRI	Gingerbread Cookie Oatmeal	Choose from snack options	Chicken Pad Thai	Choose from snack options	DINE OUT	N/A
SAT	Breakfast Sweet Potato P109	Choose from snack options	FAST FOOD MACRO GUIDE	Choose from snack options	Italian Calzones P163	*Choose from snack options
SUN	Breakfast Sweet Potato	Choose from snack options	Italian Calzones	Choose from snack options	Best Ever Chili P165	*Choose from snack options

*Be sure this snack fits into your daily calorie allotment.

WEEK 3 GROCERY LIST | Serves 2 adults for the week

PRODUCE
Asparagus, 24 spears
Avocado, 3
Bean Sprouts, 2 cups
Bell Pepper, Green, 2
Bell Pepper, Red, 2
Broccoli, 1 cup
Carrots, Matchstick, 1 cup
Cilantro, 1 bunch
Garlic, 3 cloves
Green Onions, 1 bunch
Jalapeno, 1, optional
Lemon, 1
Lettuce, Green Leaf, 8 cups
Limes, 2
Mushrooms, 1 ¼ cups
Onion, Yellow, 3
Parsley, 1 bunch
Spinach, 4 cups
Sugar Snap Peas, 1 cup
Sweet Potatoes, 1 ⅓ lb.
Tomatoes, Vine, 2
Zucchini, 2

MEAT & SEAFOOD
Beef, Lean Ground, 18 oz. (~1 lb.)
Chicken Breast, 32 oz. (2 lbs.)
Salmon, Wild Caught, 12 oz. (¾ lb.)
Turkey Bacon, 4 slices

REFRIGERATED
Cheese, Mexican, Shredded, ¼ cup
Cheese, Mozzarella, Shredded, 1 cup
Cheese, Ricotta, Part Skim, ⅓ cup
Eggs, 13
Egg Whites, 16 (2 cups liquid)
Greek Yogurt, Plain, Nonfat, ¾ cup
Pesto Sauce, ¼ cup
Spray Whipped Cream, 1 ¼ cup

PANTRY
Beans, Black, 2 cups
Beans, Kidney, 1 cup
Cashews, ¼ cup
Coconut Aminos, or Soy Sauce, 6 Tbs.

Coconut Oil, 2 Tbs.
CSE Simply Vanilla Protein Powder, 5
   servings
Honey, Raw, 2 Tbs.
Kodiak Cakes Buttermilk Mix, 1 ½ cups
Marinara Sauce, ½ cup
Molasses, 1 ¼ cup
Oats, Old-Fashioned Rolled, 3 ⅓ cups
OffBeat Gingerbread Cookie Butter
   or Almond Butter, Natural, 10 Tbs.
OffBeat Sweet Classic Peanut Butter
   or Peanut Butter, Natural, ¼ cup
Olive Oil, 2 Tbs.
Pad Thai Brown Rice Noodles, 4 oz.
   uncooked
Peanuts, 1 oz.
Rice, White, Jasmine, ½ cup uncooked
Salsa, ½ cup
Spaghetti, Whole Wheat, 5 oz.
   uncooked
Tomato Sauce, 1 cup
Tomatoes, Diced, Canned, 2 cups
Vinegar, Rice, ¼ cup
Water Chestnuts, 1 cup

SWEETENERS, SEASONINGS & SPICES
Black Pepper
Chili Powder, 2 tsp.
Cinnamon, Ground, 2 ½ tsp.
Cumin, Ground, 1 tsp.
Ginger, Ground, dash
Italian Seasoning, dash
Nutmeg, Ground, dash, optional
Oregano, Dried, ½ tsp.
Sea Salt
Taco Seasoning, 2 Tbs.

FREEZER
Corn, Yellow, 1 cup

MISC.
Cooking Spray
Parchment Paper

Remember to purchase ingredients for your selected weekly snacks!

WEEK 4

MENU PLANNER

	BREAKFAST	SNACK	LUNCH	SNACK	DINNER	*SNACK
MON	Oatmeal Cookie Shake P111	Choose from snack options	Best Ever Chili P165	Choose from snack options	California Club Tortilla Pizza P167	*Choose from snack options
TUES	Oatmeal Cookie Shake	Choose from snack options	California Club Tortilla Pizza	Choose from snack options	Black Bean & Roasted Butternut Tacos P169	*Choose from snack options
WED	Oatmeal Cookie Shake	Choose from snack options	Black Bean & Roasted Butternut Tacos	Choose from snack options	Pepper Jack Chicken Wrapped Asparagus P171	*Choose from snack options
THURS	Oatmeal Cookie Shake	Choose from snack options	Pepper Jack Chicken Wrapped Asparagus	Choose from snack options	Hearty Tuna Casserole P173	*Choose from snack options
FRI	Oatmeal Cookie Shake	Choose from snack options	Hearty Tuna Casserole	Choose from snack options	DINE OUT	N/A
SAT	Lemon Chia Pancakes P113	Choose from snack options	FAST FOOD MACRO GUIDE	Choose from snack options	Cashew Kung Pao Chicken P175	*Choose from snack options
SUN	Lemon Chia Pancakes	Choose from snack options	Cashew Kung Pao Chicken	Choose from snack options	Meatballs & Mashed Potaotes P177	*Choose from snack options

*Be sure this snack fits into your daily calorie allotment.

WEEK 4 GROCERY LIST | Serves 2 adults for the week

PRODUCE
Asparagus, 36 spears
Avocado, 2
Basil, Fresh, 1 bunch
Bell Peppers, Red, 1
Broccoli, 2 cups
Butternut Squash, Cubed, ½ cup
Cauliflower, 4 cups
Chives, 1 bunch
Cilantro, 1 bunch
Garlic, 3 cloves
Green Onions, 1 bunch
Lemon, 1
Lime, 1
Mushrooms, 1 cup
Onion, Red, 1
Onion, Yellow, 1
Potatoes, Petite Gold, ¾ lb.
Spring Salad Mix, 4 cups
Sweet Potatoes, 17 oz. (~1 lb.)
Tomatoes, Vine, 2

MEAT & SEAFOOD
Chicken Breast, 37 oz. (~2 ⅓ lbs.)
Turkey Bacon, 4 slices
Turkey, Lean, Ground, 12 oz. (¾ lb.)

REFRIGERATED
Almond Milk, Unsweetened, 5 ½ cups
Butter, Grass-Fed, 3 Tbs.
Cheese, Mozzarella, Shredded, 2 cups
Cheese, Parmesan, 2 Tbs.
Cheese, Pepper Jack, 6 slices
Cottage Cheese, Low-fat, 3 ⅓ cups
Eggs, 4
Greek Yogurt, Plain, Nonfat, 1 ¾ cups

PANTRY
Beans, Black, ½ cup
Cashews, 3 oz.
Chia Seeds, 1 ½ Tbs.
Chicken Broth, ½ cup
Coconut Aminos or Soy Sauce, 4 Tbs.
Coconut Oil, 4 tsp.
CSE Simply Vanilla Protein Powder, 5 servings
CSE Vanilla Pancake & Waffle Mix, 1 ¾ cups
Honey, Raw, 2 Tbs.
Mayo, Low-Fat, ¼ cup
Mayo, Olive Oil, 2 Tbs.
Mustard, Dijon, 5 Tbs.
Oats, Old-Fashioned Rolled, 3 ⅓ cups
OffBeat Cinnamon Bun Butter, OffBeat Gingerbread Cookie Butter or Almond Butter, Natural, 7 Tbs.
Pasta, Fusilli, Whole Grain, 5 oz. uncooked
Raisins, 50g (~⅓ cup)
Rice, White, Jasmine, ⅓ cup uncooked
Sesame Oil, ½ tsp.
Sriracha Sauce, 1 tsp.
Stubb's Original BBQ Sauce, ½ cup
Tortillas, Corn, 8
Tuna, Canned, 10 oz.
Zero Calorie Syrup of Choice, ½ cup

SWEETENERS, SEASONINGS & SPICES
All-Purpose Seasoning, dash
Black Pepper
Butter Extract, 2 tsp.
Cinnamon, 10 tsp.
Cumin, Ground, dash
Garlic Powder, 1 tsp.
Ginger, Ground, dash
Paprika, dash
Sea Salt
Stevia, Liquid Drops, Vanilla, optional

FREEZER
Ezekiel Bread, 1 slice
Tortillas, Brown Rice, 4

MISC.
Cooking Spray
Parchment Paper

Remember to purchase ingredients for your selected weekly snacks!

	BREAKFAST	SNACK	LUNCH	SNACK	DINNER	*SNACK
MON	Chocolate Peanut Butter Cup Oatmeal P115	Choose from snack options	Meatballs & Mashed Potaotes P177	Choose from snack options	Orange Almond Chicken Salad P179	*Choose from snack options
TUES	Chocolate Peanut Butter Cup Oatmeal	Choose from snack options	Orange Almond Chicken Salad	Choose from snack options	Mexican Tortilla Pizza P181	*Choose from snack options
WED	Chocolate Peanut Butter Cup Oatmeal	Choose from snack options	Mexican Tortilla Pizza	Choose from snack options	Spaghetti Squash & Bacon Fritters P183	*Choose from snack options
THURS	Chocolate Peanut Butter Cup Oatmeal	Choose from snack options	Spaghetti Squash & Bacon Fritters	Choose from snack options	Roasted Butternut Squash & Quinoa Salad P185	*Choose from snack options
FRI	Chocolate Peanut Butter Cup Oatmeal	Choose from snack options	Roasted Butternut Squash & Quinoa Salad	Choose from snack options	DINE OUT	N/A
SAT	Savory Stuffed Waffles P117	Choose from snack options	FAST FOOD MACRO GUIDE	Choose from snack options	Pepper Jack Bison Burgers P187	*Choose from snack options
SUN	Savory Stuffed Waffles	Choose from snack options	Pepper Jack Bison Burgers	Choose from snack options	Mustard Roasted Chicken & Veggies P189	*Choose from snack options

*Be sure this snack fits into your daily calorie allotment.

WEEK 5 GROCERY LIST | Serves 2 adults for the week

PRODUCE
Butternut Squash, Cubed, 1 ¼ lbs.
Carrots, ½ lb.
Chives, 1 bunch
Clementine Oranges, 4
Green Onions, 1 bunch
Lemon, 1
Lettuce, Butter, 1 head
Lettuce, Shredded, 4 cups
Onion, Red, 2
Onion, Sweet, 1
Pomegranate, 1 or Pomegranate
    Seeds, 1 cup
Spaghetti Squash, 1
Spinach, 6 cups
Spring Lettuce Mix, 8 cups
Sweet Potatoes, 1 lb.
Thyme, Fresh, 1 bunch
Tomatoes, Vine, 3
Turnips, ½ lb.

MEAT & SEAFOOD
Beef, Lean, Ground, 10 oz. (~⅔ lb.)
Bison, Lean, Ground, 12 oz. (¾ lb.)
Chicken Breast, 14 oz. (~1 lb.)
Chicken Sausage, Large (160 cals each)
    (Aidells, Coleman, Simple Truth), 2
    links
Chicken Tenderloins, 12 oz. (¾ lb.)
Turkey Bacon, 14 slices

REFRIGERATED
Cheese, Mozzarella, Shredded, 1 ½ cups
Cheese, Parmesan, Grated, 1 cup
Cheese, Pepper Jack, Shredded, 2 oz.
Eggs, 8
Egg whites, 2 cups
Greek Yogurt, Plain, Nonfat, ½ cup
Simply Orange Juice, ½ cup

PANTRY
Almonds, ¼ cup
Bread Crumbs, Whole Wheat, ¼ cup

Chocolate Chips, Extra Dark, 150 chips
Coconut Aminos or Soy Sauce, 1 Tbs.
Crackers, Sweet Potato, 24 total
Cranberries, Dried, Unsweetened,
    4 Tbs.
CSE Brownie Batter or Chocolate
    Peanut Butter Protein Powder, 5
    servings
CSE Vanilla Pancake & Waffle Mix, 2
    cups
Honey, Raw, 1 Tbs.
Ketchup, 4 Tbs.
Kodiak Cakes Buttermilk Mix, ⅔ cups
Mustard, Dijon, 1 Tbs.
Mustard, Whole Grain, 2 Tbs.
Mustard, Yellow, optional
Oats, Old-Fashioned Rolled, 5 cups
OffBeat Sweet Classic Peanut Butter
    or Peanut Butter, Natural, ¾ cup
Olive Oil, 5 Tbs.
Peanut Butter, Powdered, 1 ¼ cups
Pickles, Dill, 4
Quinoa, ⅓ cup uncooked
Salsa, ¾ cup
Vinegar, Balsamic, 2 Tbs.
Whole Wheat Hamburger Buns,
    4 (140 cals)
Zero Calorie Syrup of Choice, Optional

SWEETENERS, SEASONINGS & SPICES
All-Purpose Seasoning, dash
Black Pepper
Sea Salt
Stevia in the Raw, to taste
Taco Seasoning, 3 Tbs.

FREEZER
Tortillas, Brown Rice, 4

MISC.
Cooking Spray
Parchment Paper

Remember to purchase ingredients for your selected weekly snacks!

WEEK 6

MENU PLANNER

	BREAKFAST	SNACK	LUNCH	SNACK	DINNER	*SNACK
MON	Chocolate Chip Almond Mocha Shake P119	Choose from snack options	Mustard Roasted Chicken & Veggies P189	Choose from snack options	Lemon Pepper Chicken Salad P191	*Choose from snack options
TUES	Chocolate Chip Almond Mocha Shake	Choose from snack options	Lemon Pepper Chicken Salad	Choose from snack options	Waffled Navajo Taco P193	*Choose from snack options
WED	Chocolate Chip Almond Mocha Shake	Choose from snack options	Waffled Navajo Taco	Choose from snack options	Tomato Butter Chicken Spaghetti P195	*Choose from snack options
THURS	Chocolate Chip Almond Mocha Shake	Choose from snack options	Tomato Butter Chicken Spaghetti	Choose from snack options	Honey Garlic Salmon P197	*Choose from snack options
FRI	Chocolate Chip Almond Mocha Shake	Choose from snack options	Honey Garlic Salmon	Choose from snack options	DINE OUT	N/A
SAT	Silver Dollar Gingerbread Pancakes P121	Choose from snack options	FAST FOOD MACRO GUIDE	Choose from snack options	Spaghetti Pizza Pie P199	*Choose from snack options
SUN	Silver Dollar Gingerbread Pancakes	Choose from snack options	Spaghetti Pizza Pie	Choose from snack options	Roasted Cauliflower Soup P201	*Choose from snack options

*Be sure this snack fits into your daily calorie allotment.

WEEK 6 GROCERY LIST | Serves 2 adults for the week

PRODUCE
Avocado, 1
Bananas, 10
Basil, Fresh, 1 bunch
Broccoli, 4 cups
Brussels Sprouts, 4 cups
Cauliflower, 4 cups
Chives, Fresh, 1 bunch
Garlic, 3 cloves
Green Onions, 1 bunch
Lemons, 2
Lettuce, Green Leaf, 4 cups
Onion, Red, 1
Onion, Yellow, 1
Parsley, 1 bunch, optional
Spinach, 9 cups
Sweet Potatoes, 1 lb.
Tomatoes, Cherry, 2 cups
Tomatoes, Vine, 4

MEAT & SEAFOOD
Beef, Lean, Ground, 8 oz. (½ lb.)
Chicken Breast, 22 oz. (~1 ⅓ lb.)
Salmon, Wild Caught, 12 oz. (¾ lb.)
Turkey, Lean, Ground, 8 oz. (½ lb.)
Turkey Bacon, 4 slices

REFRIGERATED
Almond Milk, Unsweetened, 41 oz.
  (~5 ¼ cups)
Butter, Grass-Fed, 2 Tbs.
Cheese, Feta, Crumbles, ¼ cup
Cheese, Mozzarella, Shredded, 1 ½ cups
Cottage Cheese, Low-fat, ½ cup
Eggs, 15
Greek Yogurt, Plain, Nonfat, 2 ¼ cups

PANTRY
Beans, Black, ½ cup
Chicken Broth, 2 cups
Chocolate Chips, Extra Dark, 150 chips
Crio Bru or Coffee Grounds, 10 Tbs.

CSE Brownie Batter Protein,
  7 ½ servings
CSE Simply Vanilla Protein Powder,
  ½ serving
CSE Vanilla Pancake & Waffle Mix, 1 cup
Honey, Raw, 7 Tbs.
Kodiak Cakes Buttermilk Mix, 1 ½ cups
Marinara Sauce, 1 cup
Molasses, 3 Tbs.
OffBeat Almond Mocha Butter or
  Natural Almond Butter, 10 Tbs.
OffBeat Gingerbread Cookie
  Butter, OffBeat Salted Caramel
  Butter, or Natural Almond Butter,
  1 Tbs.
Olive Oil, 7 ½ Tbs.
Olives, 2 Tbs.
Salsa, ¼ cup
Spaghetti, Whole Grain, 9.5 oz.
  uncooked
Sriracha Sauce, dash, optional
White Whole-Wheat Flour, 4 cups
Yeast, Quick Rise, 1 ½ Tbs.

SWEETENERS, SEASONINGS & SPICES
Almond Extract, 2 ½ Tbs., optional
Black Pepper
Cinnamon, Ground, ½ tsp.
Ginger, Ground, ⅛ tsp.
Lemon Pepper, ¼ tsp.
Sea Salt
Taco Seasoning, 2 Tbs.
Thyme, Dried, ¼ tsp.

MISC.
Cooking Spray
Parchment Paper

Remember to purchase ingredients for your selected weekly snacks!

WEEK 7

MENU PLANNER

	BREAKFAST	SNACK	LUNCH	SNACK	DINNER	*SNACK
MON	Almond Joy Oatmeal P123	Choose from snack options	Roasted Cauliflower Soup P201	Choose from snack options	Boss Baked Mac & Cheese P203	*Choose from snack options
TUES	Almond Joy Oatmeal	Choose from snack options	Boss Baked Mac & Cheese	Choose from snack options	Supreme Pizza Popovers P205	*Choose from snack options
WED	Almond Joy Oatmeal	Choose from snack options	Supreme Pizza Popovers	Choose from snack options	Creamy Chicken Noodle Soup P207	*Choose from snack options
THURS	Almond Joy Oatmeal	Choose from snack options	Creamy Chicken Noodle Soup	Choose from snack options	Meatball Subs P209	*Choose from snack options
FRI	Almond Joy Oatmeal	Choose from snack options	Meatball Subs	Choose from snack options	DINE OUT	N/A
SAT	Chocolate Glazed Banana Crepes P125	Choose from snack options	FAST FOOD MACRO GUIDE	Choose from snack options	Thai Crunch Burger P211	*Choose from snack options
SUN	Chocolate Glazed Banana Crepes	Choose from snack options	Thai Crunch Burger	Choose from snack options	Cincinnati Style Chili P213	*Choose from snack options

***Be sure this snack fits into your daily calorie allotment.**

WEEK 7 GROCERY LIST | Serves 2 adults for the week

PRODUCE
Banana, 1
Bell Pepper, Green, 1
Bell Peppers, Red, 1
Carrots, 4
Cauliflower Florets, 3 cups
Celery Sticks, 2
Coleslaw Mix (without dressing), 4 cups
Cucumber, 1
Garlic, 4 cloves
Ginger, Fresh, 1 tsp.
Kale, 1 cup
Lemon, 1
Mushrooms, 1 cup
Onion, Red, 1
Onions, Yellow, 2
Parsley, 1 bunch
Spaghetti Squash, 1
Spinach, 1 cup

MEAT & SEAFOOD
Beef, Lean, Ground, 10 oz. (~⅔ lb.)
Chicken Sausage, Italian, 3
Rotisserie Chicken, 1
Turkey Bacon, 2 slices
Turkey, Lean, Ground, 28 oz. (1 ¾ lb.)

REFRIGERATED
Almond Milk, Unsweetened, ¼ cup
Bolthouse Farms Classic Ranch or
    Cilantro Avocado Dressing, 2 Tbs.
Butter, Grass-Fed, 2 Tbs.
Cheese, Low-Fat, Shredded,
    Cheddar, 1 cup
Cheese, Low-Fat, Shredded,
    Mozzarella, 1 cup
Cheese, Parmesan, Grated, 6 Tbs.
Egg Whites, 24 (3 cups liquid)
Eggs, 1
Greek Yogurt, Plain, Nonfat, ½ cup
Milk, Fat-Free, 2 cups

PANTRY
Baking Chocolate, Unsweetened, ¼ oz.
Beans, Kidney, 2 cups
Chicken Broth, 3 cups
Chocolate Chips, Dark, 100g
Cocoa Powder, 1 Tbs.
Coconut Aminos or Soy Sauce, 1 tsp.
Coconut Flakes, Unsweetened, ¼ cup
Coconut Milk, Lite, Canned, ¼ cup
Coconut Oil, 2 Tbs.

CSE Brownie Batter Protein,
    8 ½ servings
CSE Vanilla Pancake & Waffle Mix, 1 cup
Flour, Self-Rising, 1 cup
Honey, Raw, 3 Tbs.
Kodiak Cakes Buttermilk Mix, ¼ cups
Marinara Sauce, 1 cup
Oats, Old-Fashioned Rolled, 3 ⅓ cups
OffBeat Midnight Almond Coconut
    Butter or Almond Butter, Natural, 5 Tbs.
OffBeat Midnight Almond Coconut
    Butter or Peanut Butter, Natural, 2 Tbs.
OffBeat Sweet Classic Peanut Butter
    or Peanut Butter, Natural, 1 Tbs.
Olive Oil, 1 ½ Tbs.
Olives, Black, Sliced, Canned, ¼ cup
Pasta, Egg Noodles, 4 oz. uncooked
Pasta, Whole Wheat Macaroni or
    Elbow, 4 oz. uncooked
Pizza Sauce, Traditional, ½ cup
Tomato Paste, 1 Tbs.
Tomato Sauce, ½ cup
Vinegar, Rice, 1 tsp.
Vinegar, White Wine, ½ Tbs.
Whole-Wheat Hamburger Buns, 4
    (140 cals)
Whole-Wheat (or Potato) Hotdog Buns,
    4 (120 cals)
Worcestershire Sauce, ½ tsp.

SWEETENERS, SEASONINGS & SPICES
All-Purpose Seasoning, 1 tsp.
Bay Leaf, 2
Black Pepper
Cayenne Pepper, dash
Chili Powder, 1 Tbs.
Cinnamon, Ground, ¼ tsp.
Cloves, Ground, dash
Cumin, Ground, ¼ tsp.
Fennel Seeds, pinch
Garlic Powder, dash
Italian Seasoning, Dried, ½ tsp.
Onion, Minced, Dried, 1 ½ Tbs.
Paprika, ¼ tsp.
Parsley, Dried, ¼ tsp.
Red Pepper Flakes, pinch
Sea Salt
Stevia in the Raw, optional
Thyme, Dried, 1 tsp.

FREEZER
Ezekiel Bread, 2 slices

Remember to purchase ingredients for your selected weekly snacks!

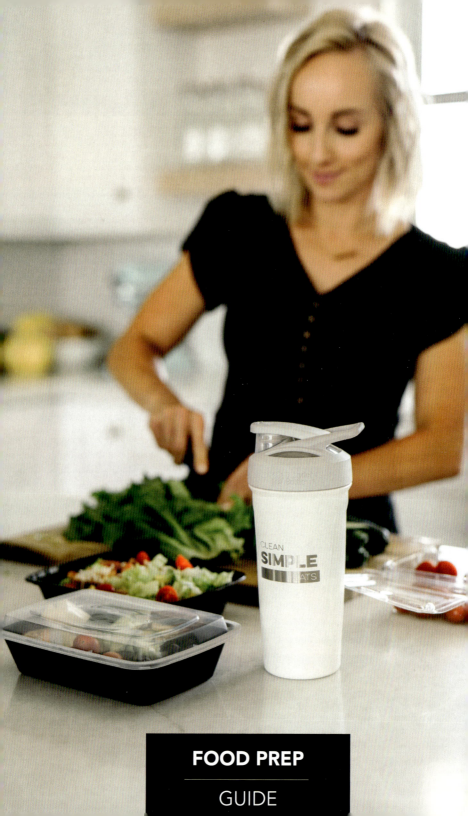

FOOD PREP

GUIDE

WEEK 1 MEAL PREP

SUNDAY PREP
- Prepare daily snacks, if needed.
- Thaw 8 oz. chicken in the fridge for the Buffalo Chicken & Pesto Sandwiches.
- Thaw 12 oz. ground beef in the fridge for the Pasta E Fagioli.
- Cook pasta and chop veggies for the Pasta E Fagioli, then store in the fridge.
- Prepare Cashew Sour Cream for Rotisserie Chicken Tacos, then store in the fridge.
- Cook 10.6 oz. chicken for the BBQ Chicken Chopped Salad.

THURSDAY PREP
- Prepare daily snacks, if needed.
- Thaw 14 oz. chicken in the fridge for the Aloha Chicken Kabobs.
- Chop veggies and pineapple for the Aloha Chicken Kabobs, then store in the fridge.
- Cook rice and prepare marinade for the Aloha Chicken Kabobs.
- Cook pasta for the Cheesy Broccoli & Penne. Add olive oil, then store in the fridge.
- Chop and cook turkey bacon for the Cheesy Broccoli & Penne, then store in the fridge.
- Thaw 9 oz. chicken tenderloins in the fridge for the Parmesan Chicken.

WEEK 2 MEAL PREP

SUNDAY PREP
- Prepare daily snacks, if needed.
- Prepare marinade/dressing for the Balsamic Chicken Chopped Salad, then store in the fridge.
- Thaw and marinate 12 oz. chicken in the fridge for the Balsamic Chicken Chopped Salad.
- Thaw and marinate 12 oz. salmon in the fridge for the Citrus Salmon Tacos.
- Chop veggies and sausage and store in the fridge for the Roasted Winter Squash & Sausage.

THURSDAY PREP
- Prepare daily snacks, if needed.
- Cook sweet potatoes and turkey bacon for the Sweet Potato Pie, then store in the fridge.
- Thaw 10 oz. chicken in the fridge for the Mexican Fajita Bowl.
- Slice veggies for the Mexican Fajita Bowl, then store in the fridge.
- Cook rice for the Mexican Fajita Bowl, then store in the fridge.
- Cook 8 oz. chicken for the Pesto Tomato & Broccoli Fusilli, then store in the fridge.
- Cook pasta for the Pesto Tomato & Broccoli Fusilli, then store in the fridge.

WEEK 3 MEAL PREP

SUNDAY PREP
- Prepare daily snacks, if needed.
- Thaw 14 oz. chicken in the fridge for the Chicken Stir-Fry.
- Cook rice for the Chicken Stir-Fry, then store in the fridge.
- Thaw 10 oz. lean ground beef in the fridge for the Taco Salad.
- Thaw salmon in the fridge for the Salmon & Greens Spaghetti.
- Spiralize zucchini for the Salmon & Greens Spaghetti, then store in the fridge.

THURSDAY PREP
- Prepare daily snacks, if needed.
- Thaw 11 oz. chicken in the fridge for the Chicken Pad Thai.
- Prepare the peanut butter sauce for the Chicken Pad Thai, then store in the fridge.
- Cook and shred 5 oz. chicken for the Italian Calzones, then store in the fridge.
- Thaw 8 oz. lean ground beef in the fridge for the Best Ever Chili.

WEEK 4 MEAL PREP

SUNDAY PREP
- Prepare daily snacks, if needed.
- Cook turkey bacon for the California Club Tortilla Pizza.
- Cook 15 oz. chicken for the Black Bean & Roasted Butternut Tacos and the California Club Tortilla Pizza, then store in the fridge.
- Roast butternut squash for the Black Bean & Roasted Butternut Tacos, then store in the fridge.
- Thaw 10 oz. chicken in the fridge for the Pepper Jack Chicken Wrapped Asparagus.

THURSDAY PREP
- Prepare daily snacks, if needed.
- Cook pasta for the Hearty Tuna Casserole, then store in the fridge.
- Chop veggies for the Hearty Tuna Casserole, then store in the fridge.
- Thaw 12 oz. chicken in the fridge for the Cashew Kung Pao Chicken.
- Cook rice for the Cashew Kung Pao Chicken, then store in the fridge.
- Prepare the Sweet & Spicy Kung Pao Sauce for the Cashew Kung Pao Chicken, then store in the fridge.
- Thaw 8 oz. lean ground turkey in the fridge for the Meatballs & Mashed Potatoes.

WEEK 5 MEAL PREP

SUNDAY PREP
- Prepare daily snacks, if needed.
- Thaw and marinate 12 oz. chicken for the Orange Almond Chicken Salad.
- Prepare the Orange Balsamic Marinade for the Orange Almond Chicken Salad, then store in the fridge.
- Thaw and/or cook 10 oz. lean ground beef for the Mexican Tortilla Pizza.
- Chop and cook bacon for the Spaghetti Squash & Bacon Fritters, then store in the fridge.

THURSDAY PREP
- Prepare daily snacks, if needed.
- Cook quinoa for the Butternut Squash & Quinoa Salad, then store in the fridge.
- Thaw 12 oz. lean ground bison in the fridge for the Pepper Jack Bison Burgers.
- Thaw 14 oz. chicken in the fridge for the Mustard Roasted Chicken & Veggies.
- Chop veggies for the Mustard Roasted Chicken & Veggies, then store in the fridge.

WEEK 6 MEAL PREP

SUNDAY PREP
- Prepare daily snacks, if needed.
- Thaw 22 oz. chicken in the fridge for the Lemon Pepper Chicken Salad and the Tomato Butter Chicken Spaghetti.
- Thaw 8 oz. lean ground beef in the fridge for the Waffled Navajo Taco.
- Bake Homemade Honey-Wheat Bread for the Lemon Pepper Chicken Salad
- Chicken Salad and Roasted Cauliflower Soup, then cover in plastic wrap or foil.

THURSDAY PREP
- Prepare daily snacks, if needed.
- Cube and trim veggies for the Honey Garlic Salmon, then store in the fridge.
- Thaw 12 oz. salmon in the fridge for the Honey Garlic Salmon.
- Thaw 26 oz. lean ground turkey in the fridge for the Spaghetti Pizza Pie.
- Cook spaghetti for the Spaghetti Pizza Pie, then store in the fridge.

WEEK 7 MEAL PREP

SUNDAY PREP
- Prepare daily snacks, if needed.
- Slice the chicken sausage and turkey bacon for the Boss Baked Mac & Cheese, then store in a container or bag in the fridge.
- Make the breadcrumbs for the Boss Baked Mac & Cheese.
- Thaw 6 oz. lean ground turkey for the Supreme Pizza Popovers.
- Chop the carrots, celery and kale for the Creamy Chicken Noodle Soup, then store in the fridge.
- Shred the rotisserie chicken for the Creamy Chicken Noodle Soup, then store in the fridge.

THURSDAY PREP
- Prepare daily snacks, if needed.
- Make the Chocolate Glaze for the Chocolate Glazed Banana Crepes, then store in the fridge.
- Thaw 22 oz. lean ground turkey for the Meatball Subs and the Thai Crunch Burger.
- Make the breadcrumbs for the Meatball Subs.
- Chop the spinach and red bell peppers for the Meatball Subs.
- Chop the red bell peppers, the carrots and the onions for the Thai Crunch Burger.
- Prepare the Thai Peanut Dressing for the Thai Crunch Burger, then store in the fridge.
- Thaw 10 oz. lean ground beef for the Cincinnati Style Chili.

CHICKEN

GRILL (whole)
1. Preheat grill to high heat.

2. Make sure chicken is completely thawed out. Butterfly cut chicken breasts (optional, helps them cook faster).

3. Turn heat down to medium, lightly spray grill with non-stick cooking spray and place chicken on grill. Grill about 5-7 minutes per side, flipping occasionally. Chicken is done when it is no longer pink and juices run clear.

4. Season and serve warm or store in the fridge for future use. Use within 3-4 days.

BROIL (whole)
1. Preheat oven to HI broil. Move oven rack to the very top.

2. Spray broiler pan with non-stick cooking spray. Make sure chicken is completely thawed out. Butterfly cut chicken breasts (optional, helps them cook faster) and place on broiler pan.

3. Broil 7-8 minutes per side. Chicken is done when it is no longer pink and juices run clear.

4. Season and serve warm or store in the fridge for future use. Use within 3-4 days.

5. For easy shredding, place in a Kitchen Aid Mixer while warm and mix on low. Hand mixers will work as well.

CROCKPOT (soft, shredded)
1. Place chicken in crockpot with 1 cup of water, seasonings and/or low-sodium chicken stock.

2. Turn crockpot on low and cook for 5-6 hours OR on high for 3-4 hours. Chicken is done when it is no longer pink and juices run clear. Chicken should be soft and easy to shred.

3. Season and serve warm or store in the fridge for future use. Use within 3-4 days.

INSTANT POT (soft, shredded)
1. Place 2 lbs. of thawed or frozen chicken in the Instant Pot with 1 cup of water and seasonings or low-sodium chicken stock. If the chicken is frozen, make sure it is broken apart and not frozen in a big clump or it will not cook.

2. Seal lid. Press the manual button and cook on high pressure 9 minutes if thawed and 12 minutes if frozen.

3. The Instant Pot will take a few minutes to heat up and seal before it starts cooking. Let it run its course and once it's done, let it self-vent for 10 minutes. Then manually vent and remove the lid.

4. Season and serve warm or store in the fridge or freezer for future use. Keeps in the fridge 4-5 days and the freezer one month.

SKILLET (cubed)
1. Heat skillet to medium heat and grease with cooking spray. Cube thawed chicken and place in skillet. Season the chicken with salt, pepper and other seasonings of choice. Cover.

2. Stir and flip every three minutes until all sides are golden brown and chicken is cooked through. Place in a sealed container and store in the fridge or freezer.

ROASTED SPAGHETTI SQUASH

1. Preheat oven to 400 degrees.

2. Cut spaghetti squash into 2-inch rings. Place on a greased baking sheet. Spray the tops of the squash with cooking spray and sprinkle with sea salt. Bake for 40 minutes, flipping halfway.

3. Let cool until you can hold in your hands. Rake squash into a bowl like spaghetti. Serve warm or store in the fridge. Use within 5-7 days.

HARD BOILED EGGS

STOVETOP
1. Place eggs in a pot and fill with water until it covers the eggs.

2. Place pot over high heat and cover. Once water comes to a boil, boil for 2 minutes then remove from heat. Keep covered for 10 minutes.

3. Drain water from pot and run cold water over the top. Transfer the eggs into a separate bowl filled with ice.

4. Once cool, place eggs in a bowl and refrigerate. Peel when ready to eat. Store in the fridge up to 2 weeks.

INSTANT POT
1. Place 6-12 eggs on the rack inside the Instant Pot. Add 1 cup of water.

2. Cook for 6 minutes on manual. Vent immediately and place eggs into a bowl filled with ice.

3. Once cool, place eggs in a bowl and refrigerate. Peel when ready to eat. Store in the fridge up to two weeks.

ROASTED SWEET POTATOES & RED POTATOES

CUBES OR FRIES
1. Preheat oven to 400 degrees. Move oven rack to the center of your oven.

2. Wash and cube or cut sweet potatoes into bite-sized pieces or fries with a sharp knife. Spread out in a single layer onto a baking sheet lined with parchment paper.

3. Spray the tops with cooking spray and sprinkle tops with sea salt and other seasonings of choice. Bake for 20 minutes, flip and bake an additional 15 minutes. Potatoes should be fork-tender.

4. Serve warm or store in the fridge. Use within 5-7 days.

WHOLE
1. Preheat oven to 400 degrees. Wash sweet potatoes and poke holes all over with a fork

or knife. Wrap in tin foil or spray with cooking spray and sprinkle with sea salt.

2. Bake for 60 minutes, flipping halfway through.

3. Serve warm or store in a bowl in the fridge. Use within 5-7 days.

ROASTED BRUSSELS

1. Preheat oven to 400 degrees.

2. Trim ends off of the Brussels sprouts and cut in half.

3. Place in a single layer on a baking sheet lined with parchment paper. Spray the tops with cooking spray. Sprinkle with sea salt. Bake for 20 minutes.

ROASTED BROCCOLI & CAULIFLOWER

1. Preheat oven to 400 degrees. Chop broccoli or cauliflower into florets. Place on a baking sheet lined with parchment paper. Spread out into a single layer and spray the tops with cooking spray. Sprinkle with sea salt and other seasonings of choice.

2. Bake 20 minutes. Serve warm or store in the fridge. Use within 5-7 days.

ROASTED ASPARAGUS

1. Preheat oven to 400 degrees.

2. Wash and trim hard, white ends off of asparagus stalks.

3. Place in a single layer on a baking sheet lined with parchment paper. Spray the tops with cooking spray. Sprinkle with sea salt. Bake for 8-10 minutes.

ROASTED BUTTERNUT SQUASH

1. Preheat oven to 350 degrees.

2. Peel and cube butternut squash. Place on a baking sheet lined with parchment paper in a single layer. Spray tops with cooking spray and sprinkle with sea salt.

3. Bake for 40 minutes, flipping halfway.

HOMEMADE HONEY-WHEAT BREAD
Makes 24 servings
105 calories / 1.5F / 22C / 4P

---

4 cups (715g) white whole wheat flour
1 ½ Tbs. quick rise yeast
1 ½ tsp. sea salt
2 cups warm water (100-115 degrees)
4 Tbs. raw honey
1 ½ Tbs. olive oil

1. Stir dry ingredients together in a bowl. Add the wet ingredients and mix for one minute. Dough should be slightly sticky. If dry, add more water. If too sticky to handle, add more flour.

2. Knead for 5 minutes using a bread mixer, kitchen aid or your hands.

3. Form dough into two balls. Place on a baking sheet lined with parchment paper. Cover with a dish towel and let rise for 25 minutes. Preheat oven to 350 degrees.

4. Score the top of each loaf with a sharp knife. Bake for 22-25 minutes or until golden brown. Remove from the oven and cool on a wire rack.

5. Weigh the bread and divide the weight by 24 to get the amount needed for one serving.

APPROVED PROTEIN BARS
Built Bars
G2G Bars
Kirkland Protein Bars
No Cow Bars
Oatmega Bars
One Bars Basix Bars (no sucralose)
Perfect Bars
Probar Base Bars
Quest Bars (no sucralose)
RX Bars
Square Bars
Vega Bars

*Visit www.cleansimpleeats.com/ blog/bars for our favorite flavors and discount codes!

CASHEW SOUR CREAM
Makes 8 servings / 1 Tbs. per serving
50 calories / 4F / 2C / 1P / per serving

½ cup unsalted cashews
1 Tbs. lemon juice
½ Tbs. olive oil
¼ tsp. sea salt
¼-½ cup water

1. Soak the cashews in water for 30+ minutes.

2. Drain the cashews and add to a high-powered blender. Add the lemon juice, olive oil, sea salt and ¼ cup water.

3. Blend on high. Add an additional ¼ cup water if the mixture is too thick. It should be a pourable consistency, but not too runny. Pour into a sealed container and store in the fridge. Use within 5-7 days.

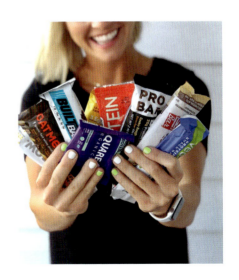

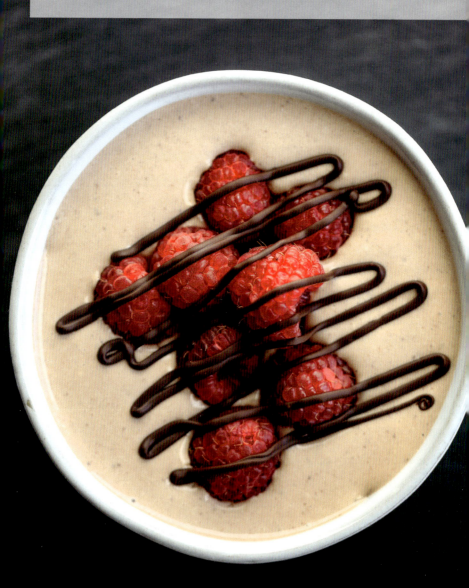

KEEP YOUR FRIENDS CLOSE AND YOUR SNACKS CLOSER

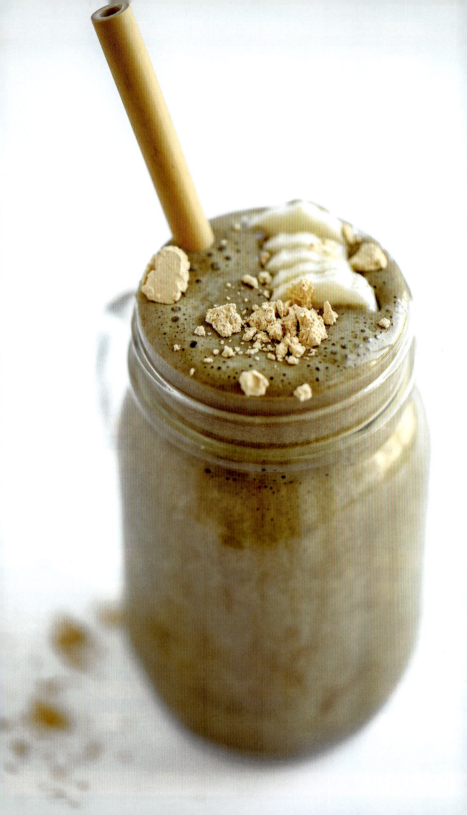

CHOCOLATE PEANUT BUTTER SHAKE

Makes 1 serving
245 calories / 7F / 25C / 20P

---

1 cup unsweetened cashew milk
½ serving (17g) CSE Brownie Batter or Chocolate Peanut
    Butter Protein Powder
½ Tbs. OffBeat Sweet Classic Peanut Butter
    or natural peanut butter
2 Tbs. powdered peanut butter
50g frozen banana slices
1 Tbs. cocoa powder
1 cup spinach
6-8 (120g) ice cubes

1. Add all of the ingredients to a high-powered blender. Blend on high until smooth.

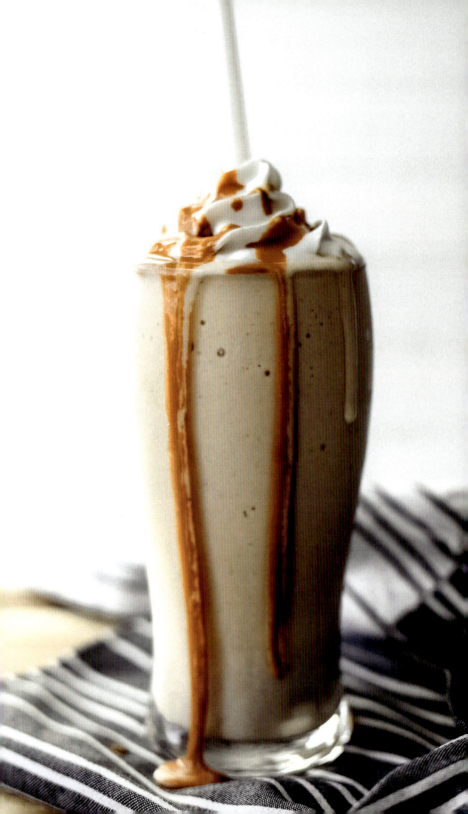

PEANUT BUTTER CARAMEL MILKSHAKE

Makes 1 serving
240 calories / 6.5F / 24C / 20.5P

½ cup fat-free milk
½ cup Halo Top Sea Salt Caramel or Vanilla Bean Ice Cream
30g frozen banana slices
2 Tbs. CSE Simply Vanilla or Caramel Toffee Protein Powder
½ Tbs. OffBeat Sweet Classic Peanut Butter
   or natural peanut butter
6-8 (120g) ice cubes

Topping:
2 Tbs. spray whipped cream topping
1 tsp. Walden Farms Caramel Syrup

1. Add all of the ingredients to a high-powered blender. Blend on high until smooth.

2. Top with whipped cream and enjoy!

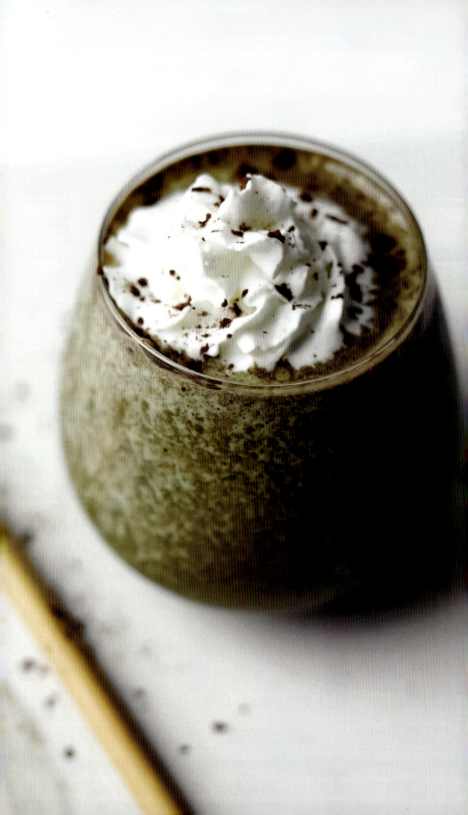

THIN MINT SHAKE
Makes 1 serving
240 calories / 9F / 24C / 15.5P

---

1 cup unsweetened almond milk
½ serving CSE Mint Chocolate Cookie or Brownie Batter
   Protein Powder
30g frozen banana slices
1 Tbs. OffBeat Mint Chocolate Chip Cookie Butter
1 Tbs. cocoa powder
1 cup spinach
6-8 (120g) ice cubes
Topping:
2 Tbs. spray whipped cream topping

1. Add all of the ingredients to a high-powered blender. Blend on high until smooth.

2. Top with whipped cream and enjoy!

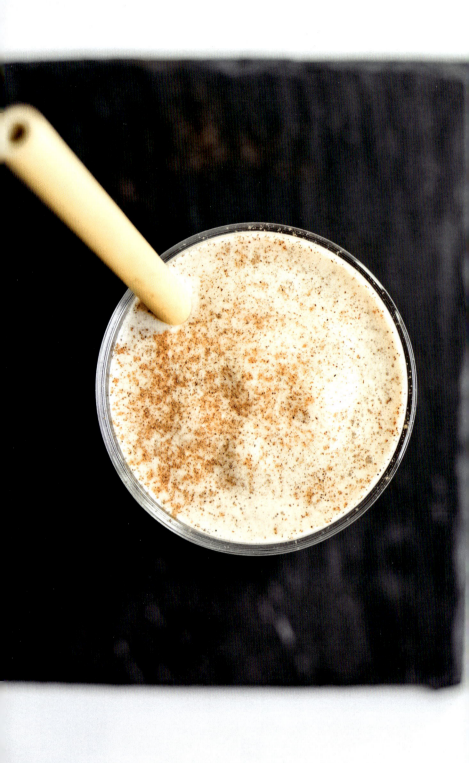

VANILLA CHAI SHAKE

Makes 1 serving
235 calories / 8.5F / 25C / 15P

1 cup unsweetened almond milk
½ serving CSE Simply Vanilla or Snickerdoodle Protein Powder
50g frozen banana slices
½ Tbs. OffBeat Cinnamon Bun Butter
   or natural almond butter
2 Tbs. old-fashioned rolled oats
1 tsp. chia seeds
1 tsp. ground cinnamon
¼ tsp. ground ginger
¼ tsp. cardamom
Dash of cloves, optional
6-8 (120g) ice cubes

1. Add all of the ingredients to a high-powered blender. Blend on high until smooth.

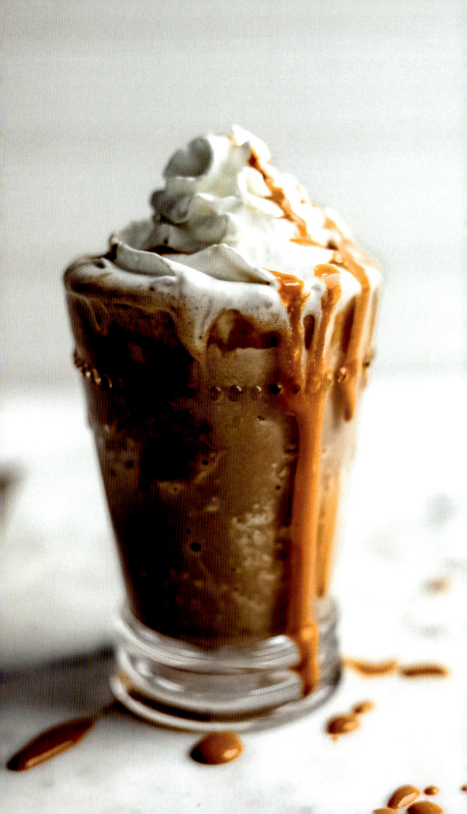

SNICKERS SHAKE

Makes 1 serving
220 calories / 7.5F / 22.5C / 16P

½ cup fat-free milk
2 Tbs. CSE Brownie Batter, Chocolate Peanut Butter
  or Caramel Toffee Protein Powder
30g frozen banana slices
1 Tbs. old-fashioned rolled oats
2 tsp. OffBeat Sweet Classic Peanut Butter, Salted Caramel
  or natural peanut butter
1 tsp. cocoa powder
6-8 (120g) ice cubes

Topping:
2 Tbs. spray whipped cream topping
Walden Farms Caramel Syrup

1. Add all of the ingredients to a high-powered blender. Blend on high until smooth.

2. Top with whipped cream and caramel syrup. Enjoy!

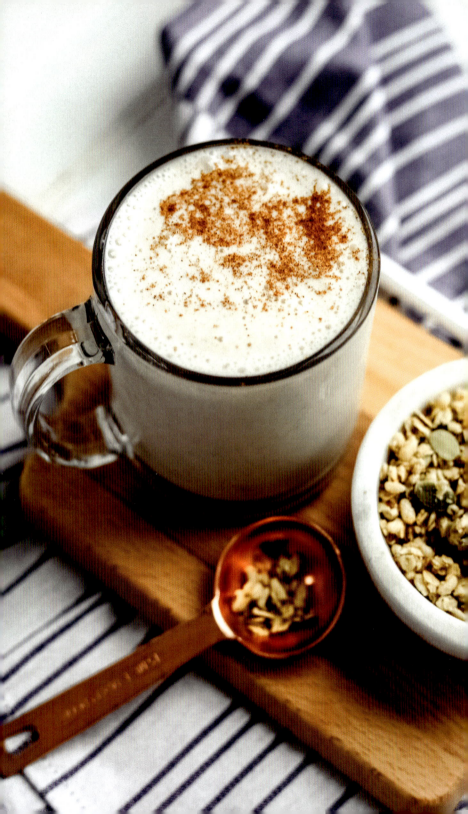

PROTEIN POWER CRUNCH SHAKE

Makes 1 serving
240 calories / 8F / 25C / 17P

---

1 cup unsweetened almond milk
½ cup low-fat cottage cheese
3 Tbs. Nature's Path Pumpkin Seed & Flax Granola
50g frozen banana slices
Dash of cinnamon
Vanilla stevia drops, optional
6-8 (120g) ice cubes

1. Add all of the ingredients to a high-powered blender. Blend on high until smooth.

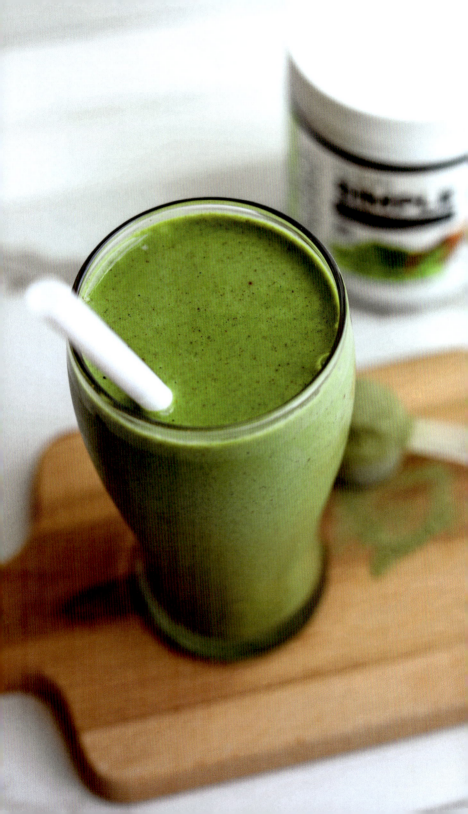

POWER GREENS SHAKE

Makes 1 serving
237 calories / 7F / 27C / 16P

---

1 cup unsweetened almond milk
¾ serving CSE Simply Vanilla Protein Powder
1 serving CSE Super Greens Mix
50g frozen banana slices
½ Tbs. OffBeat Aloha Butter, Almond Mocha Butter
   or natural almond butter
1 cup spinach
Dash of cinnamon
6-8 (120g) ice cubes

1. Add all of the ingredients to a high-powered blender. Blend on high until smooth.

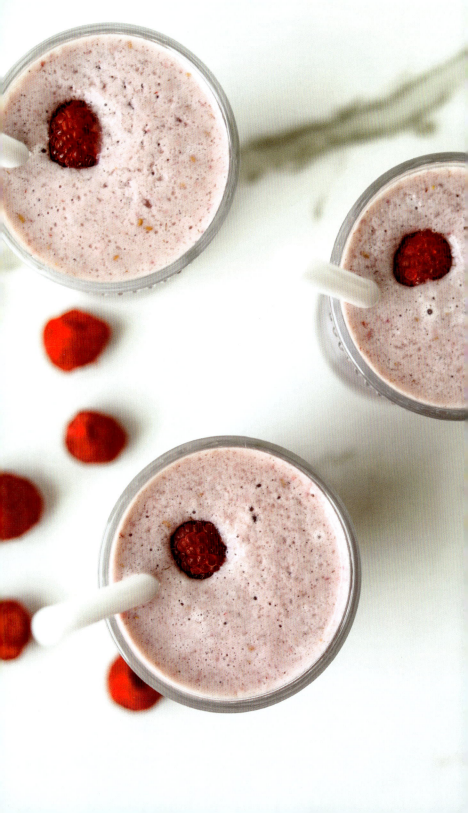

RADIANT RASPBERRY SHAKE

Makes 1 serving
185 calories / 5F / 3C / 15P

1 cup unsweetened almond milk
½ cup fresh or frozen raspberries
½ serving CSE Strawberry Cheesecake or Simply Vanilla
   Protein Powder
1 serving CSE Super Berry Mix
2 Tbs. low-fat cottage cheese
½ Tbs. OffBeat Aloha Butter, Lemon Coconut Bliss Butter
   or natural almond butter
¼ tsp. almond extract
6-8 (120g) ice cubes

1. Add all of the ingredients to a high-powered blender. Blend on
high until smooth.

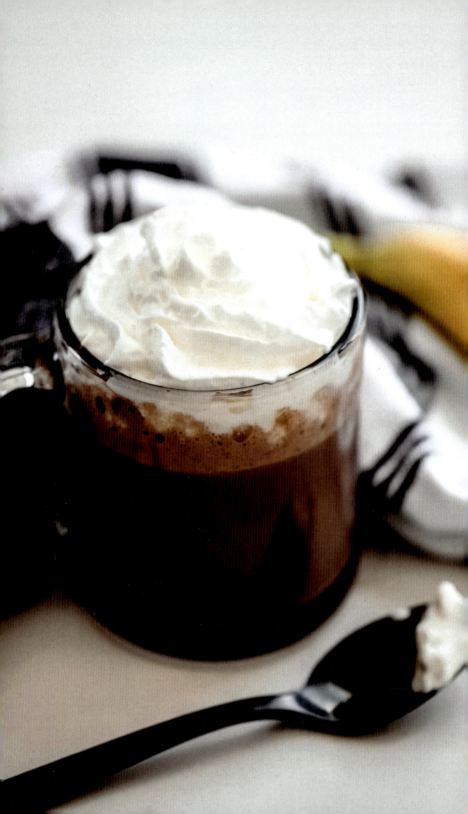

CSE HOT COCOA

Makes 1 serving
245 calories / 2F / 25.5C / 30.5P

---

1 cup water
1 ½ servings CSE Brownie Batter Protein Powder
Topping:
¼ cup spray whipped cream topping
Side:
50g of a banana

1. Add water to a mug and microwave for 1-2 minutes or until hot. Let cool for a couple minutes.

2. Add protein powder and whisk until smooth.

3. Top with whipped cream and enjoy the banana on the side.

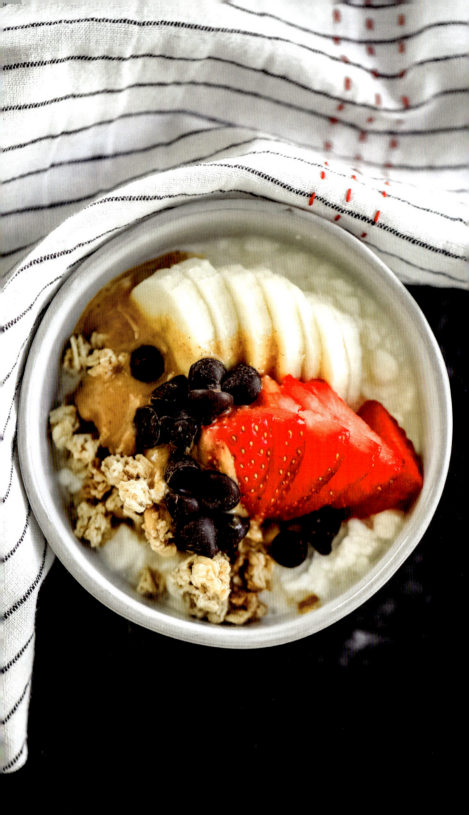

CHUNKY MONKEY BOWL

Makes 1 serving
250 calories / 10F / 23C / 17P

½ cup low-fat cottage cheese
Vanilla stevia drops
30g banana slices
1 large sliced strawberry
2 Tbs. Nature's Path Pumpkin Seed & Flax Granola
½ Tbs. OffBeat Sweet Classic Butter, Candy Bar Butter,
   Monkey Business Butter or natural peanut butter
8 (4g) dark chocolate chips

1. Combine the cottage cheese and stevia in a bowl.

2. Top with bananas, strawberries, granola, peanut butter and chocolate chips.

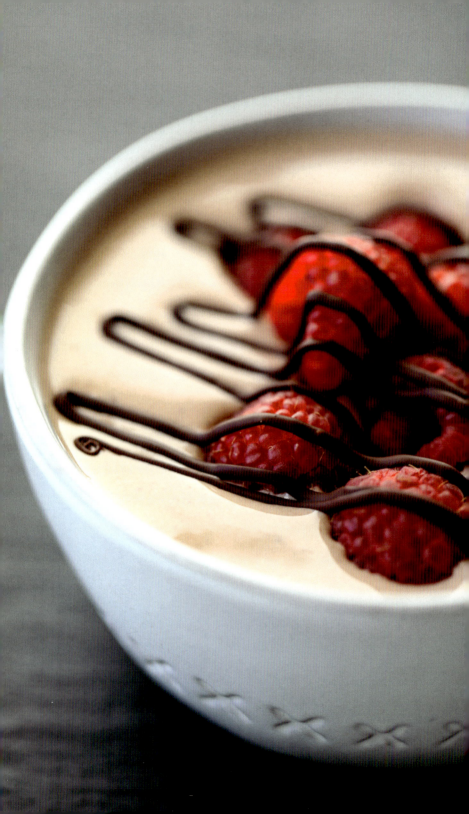

DARK CHOCOLATE MOUSSE

Makes 1 serving
250 calories / 8F / 28C / 17P

⅔ cup nonfat, plain Greek yogurt
1 Tbs. cocoa powder
1 tsp. raw honey
Vanilla stevia drops, optional
¼ cup fresh raspberries
15g dark chocolate chips, melted
2 Tbs. spray whipped cream topping

1. Stir the Greek yogurt, cocoa powder, honey and stevia together in a bowl. Add the fresh raspberries.

2. Place the chocolate chips in a bowl and heat in the microwave for 30 seconds at a time until melted and smooth; stirring in between.

3. Drizzle the chocolate over the raspberries and top with whipped cream.

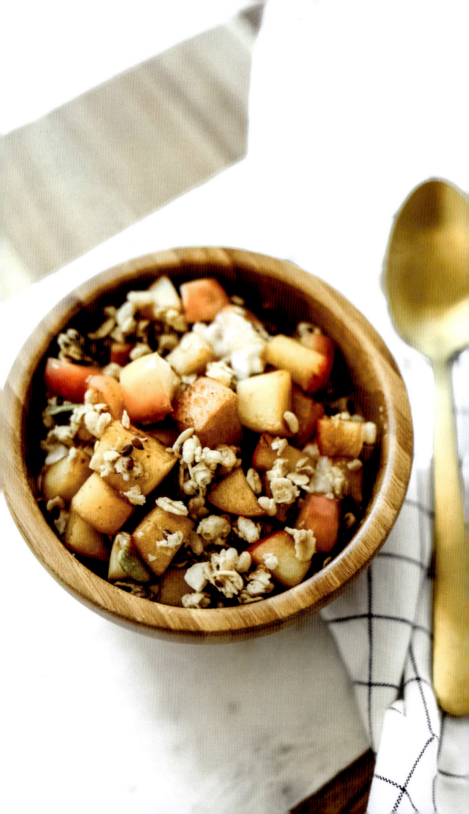

CREAMY CINNAMON SUGAR APPLE BOWL

Makes 1 serving
240 calories / 9F / 25C / 15P

½ cup low-fat cottage cheese
Vanilla stevia drops
75g chopped apple
1 tsp. coconut oil
1 tsp. coconut sugar
1 tsp. ground cinnamon
2 Tbs. Nature's Path Pumpkin Seed & Flax Granola

1. Combine the cottage cheese and stevia drops in a bowl; set aside.

2. In a frying pan over medium heat, sauté the apples in coconut oil, coconut sugar and cinnamon. Cook until fragrant.

3. Pour the apples over the cottage cheese and sprinkle granola over the top.

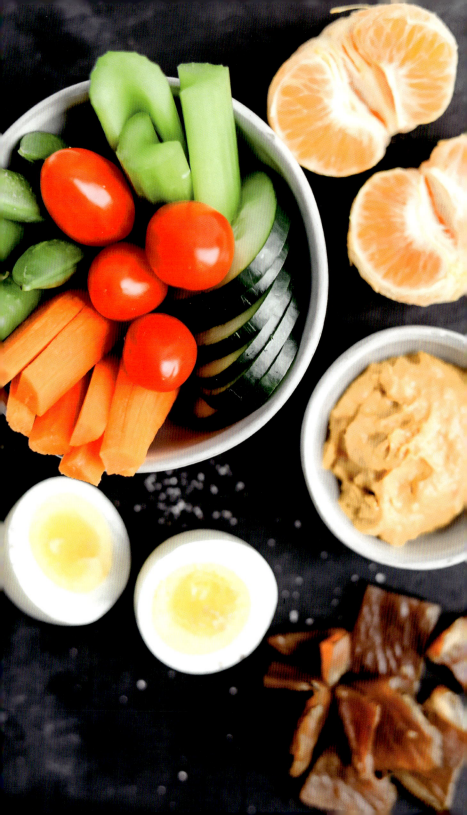

GRAB & GO SNACK

Makes 1 serving
240 calories / 8F / 24C / 18P

1 cup veggies of choice
1 Tbs. hummus
1 boiled egg
22g turkey jerky
1 clementine orange

1. Use hummus as a dip for the veggies. Enjoy boiled egg, turkey jerky and orange on the side.

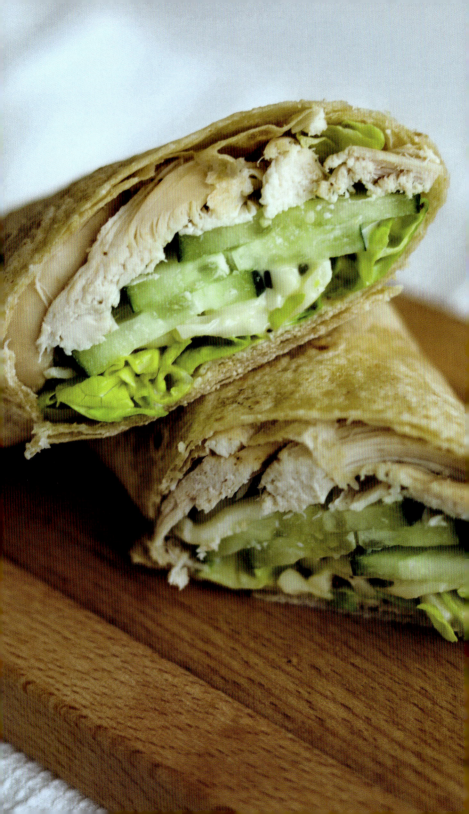

CHICKEN SNACK WRAP
Makes 1 serving
225 calories / 6F / 26C / 17P

---

1 whole grain or whole wheat tortilla (120 cals)
1.5 oz. rotisserie chicken breast
½ cup shredded lettuce
6 cucumber slices
Sea salt
Ground black pepper
1 Tbs. low-fat, shredded mozzarella cheese
2 tsp. Bolthouse Farms Honey Mustard Dressing

1. Lay out tortilla. Pile in all of the ingredients and wrap up tight.

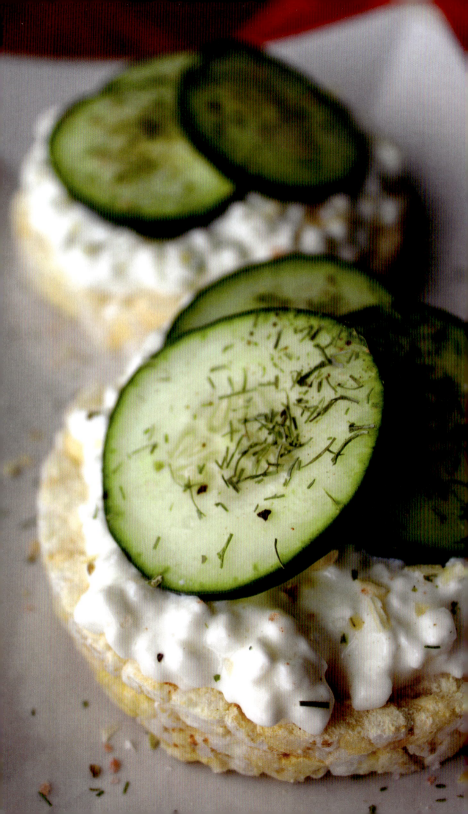

OPEN FACED CHEESE & CUCUMBERS

Makes 1 serving
240 calories / 7.5F / 25C / 18P

---

2 white cheddar rice cakes
½ cup low-fat cottage cheese
8 cucumber slices
Dried dill and minced onions
    or Trader Joe's Everything Bagel Seasoning
Sea salt and pepper, to taste
Side:
8g raw almonds

1. Top each rice cake with ¼ cup cottage cheese, 4 cucumber slices, seasoning of choice, sea salt and pepper to taste. Enjoy the almonds on the side.

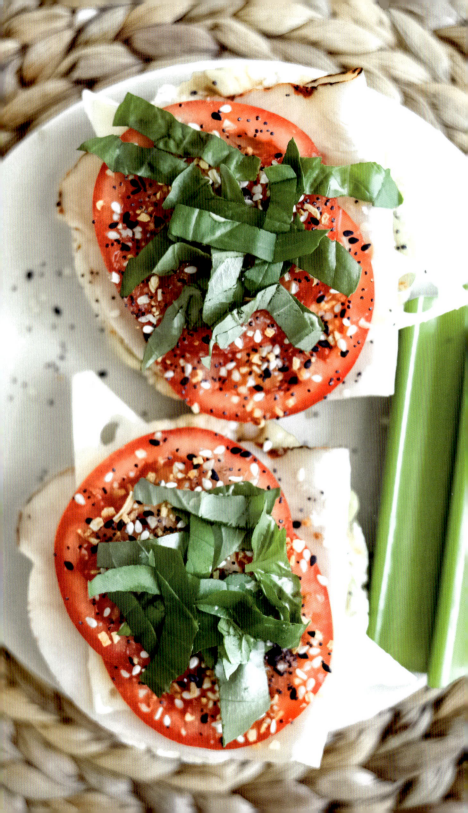

OPEN FACED TURKEY & SWISS
Makes 1 serving
230 calories / 9F / 21C / 16P

2 original or white cheddar rice cakes
1 tsp. Dijon mustard
1 oz. nitrate-free deli turkey
1 slice Swiss cheese
4 vine tomato slices
Trader Joe's Everything Bagel Seasoning
or dried minced onion
Sea salt and pepper, to taste
Fresh basil, chopped
Side:
2 celery sticks

1. Layer the rice cakes evenly with mustard, turkey, cheese and tomato slices. Sprinkle with seasonings, sea salt and pepper and fresh basil. Enjoy celery on the side.

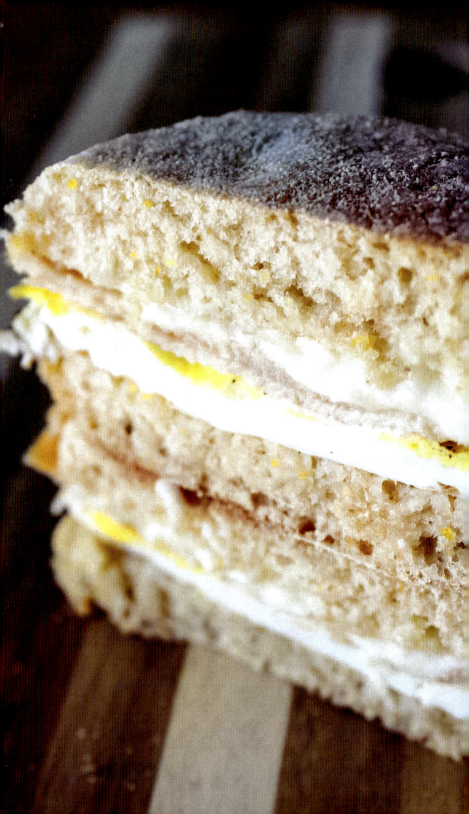

BREAKFAST SANDWICHES BY THE DOZEN

Makes 12 servings / 1 breakfast sandwich per serving
245 calories / 5F / 32C / 18P / per serving

---

6 large eggs
12 egg whites
2 Tbs. water
12 multigrain English muffins
¾ cup low-fat, shredded mozzarella cheese
12 oz. nitrate-free deli turkey

1. Preheat oven to 350 degrees.

2. Beat the eggs and egg whites with water. Spray a 9x13 pan with cooking spray. Pour the egg mixture into the pan and bake for 20 minutes. Slice into 12 equal portions.

3. Slice the English muffins in half and lay them out in a single layer. Place one egg portion on top of 12 of the halves. Add 1 ounce of deli turkey and 1 tablespoon of cheese on top of each egg portion. Sandwich with the other half of the muffin.

4. Spray a piece of foil with cooking spray. Wrap each sandwich individually in foil, place in a Ziploc freezer bag and store in the fridge or freezer.

5. Transfer to the fridge the night before eating to let thaw. When ready to eat, pop in the oven at 375 degrees for 20 minutes. If frozen, reheat in the oven for an extra 15-20 minutes. Enjoy warm.

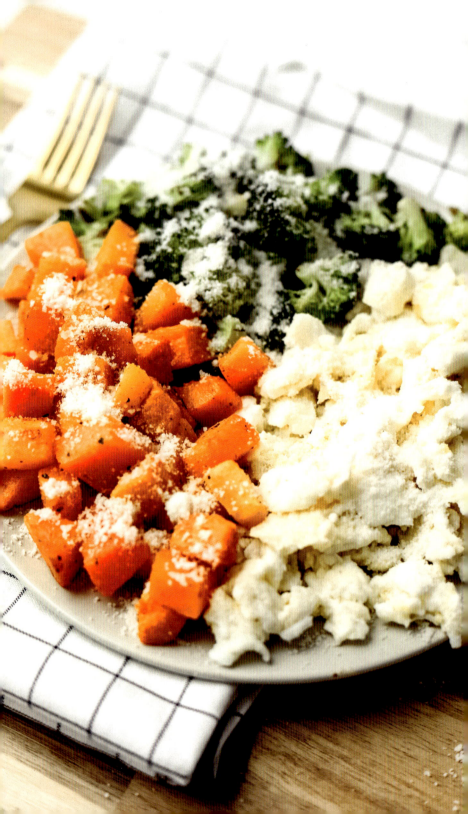

BUTTERNUT SQUASH SCRAMBLE

Makes 1 serving
230 calories / 8F / 23C / 17P

¾ cup butternut squash, diced and roasted
½ cup broccoli, diced and roasted
1 large egg
1 egg white
Sea salt and pepper, to taste
2 Tbs. grated Parmesan cheese

1. Roast the butternut squash and broccoli according to the directions in the Food Prep Guide.

2. Scramble the egg and egg white in a frying pan over medium heat. Add the roasted veggies to the pan and combine. Sprinkle with sea salt and pepper then top with cheese. Enjoy warm.

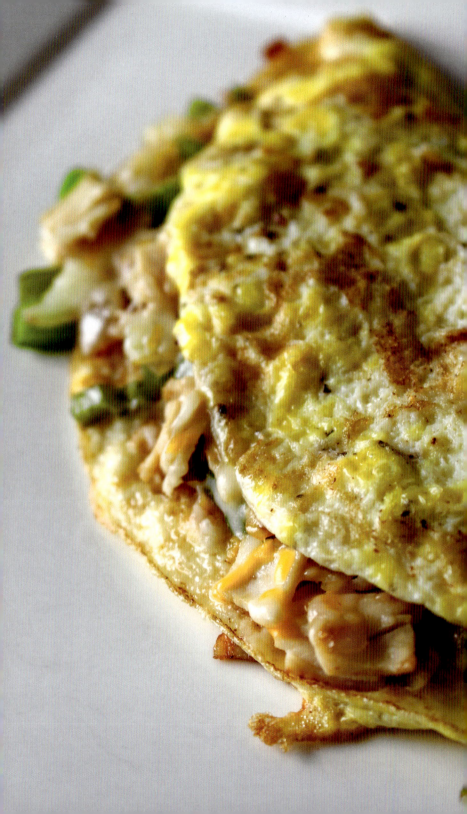

DENVER OMELET

Makes 1 serving
245 calories / 9F / 22C / 20P

2 Tbs. diced green bell pepper
2 Tbs. diced yellow onion
1 oz. diced, nitrate-free deli turkey
1 large egg
1 egg white
1 Tbs. water
2 Tbs. low-fat, shredded cheddar cheese
Sea salt and pepper, to taste
Side:
2 small clementine oranges

1. Heat a frying pan over medium heat. Spray pan and add the veggies and turkey. Sauté until veggies are tender. Remove from pan.

2. Beat the egg, egg white and water together in a bowl. Spray the pan again and add the egg mixture. Sprinkle with sea salt and pepper. Once the bottom is cooked, flip over.

3. Add the veggies and cheese to center and fold half of the fried eggs over the top creating an omelet. Once the cheese is melted, remove from pan. Enjoy warm with oranges on the side.

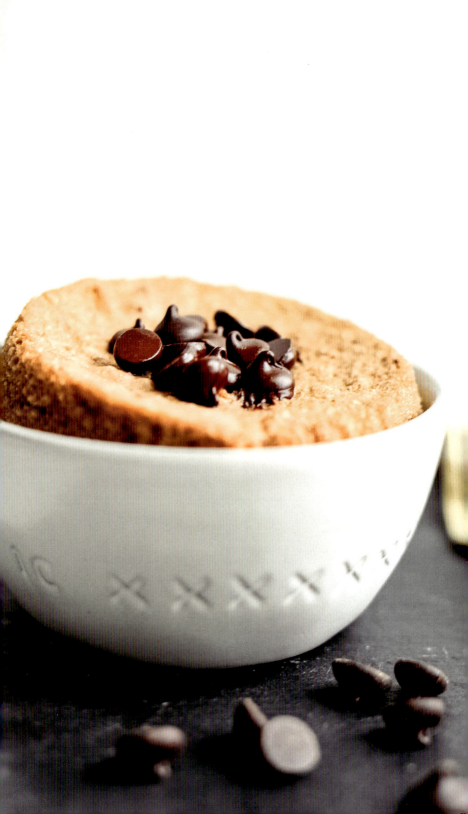

DARK CHOCOLATE MUG CAKE

Makes 1 serving
230 calories / 7F / 24C / 18P

3 Tbs. unsweetened vanilla almond milk
3 Tbs (46g) liquid egg whites
½ tsp. vanilla extract
Liquid vanilla stevia drops, to taste
⅓ cup CSE Vanilla Pancake & Waffle Mix
1 tsp. cocoa powder
10g OffBeat Midnight Almond Coconut, Buckeye Brownie Butter
   or 15g extra dark chocolate chips
Zero calorie syrup of choice, optional

1. Spray a mug or bowl with cooking spray and whisk in the almond milk, egg whites, vanilla extract and stevia. Add the CSE Pancake & Waffle Mix and cocoa powder. Whisk together until well combined.

2. Heat in the microwave for 60-90 seconds. Top with nut butter or chocolate chips. Drizzle with syrup, if desired.

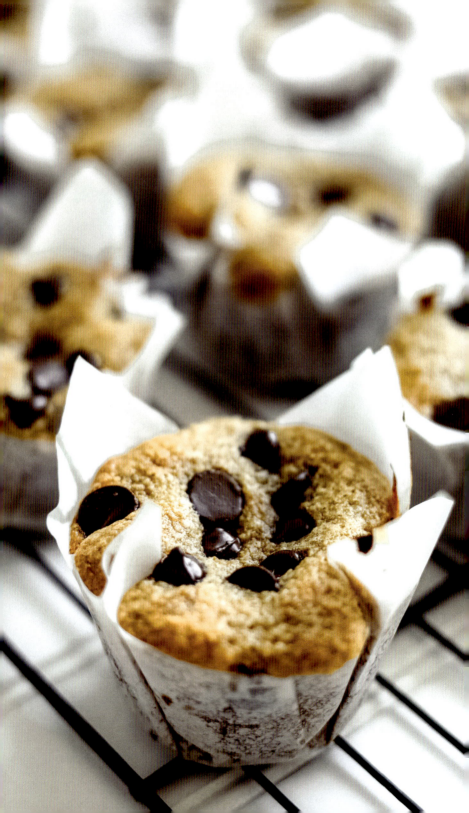

BANANA CHOCOLATE CHIP MUFFINS

Makes 13 muffins / 1 per serving
180 calories / 6.5F / 26C / 6.5P / per serving

---

2 (240g) ripe bananas
½ cup raw honey
3 Tbs. melted coconut oil
½ cup unsweetened applesauce
1 large egg
1 tsp. vanilla extract
1 ½ cups CSE Vanilla Pancake & Waffle Mix
1 serving CSE Simply Vanilla Protein Powder
2 Tbs. flaxseed meal
1 tsp. baking soda
1 tsp. baking powder
¼ tsp. sea salt

Topping per muffin:
10 dark chocolate chips (5 grams per muffin)

1. Preheat oven to 350 degrees.

2. Mash the bananas in a large mixing bowl. Beat in the honey and coconut oil. Add in the applesauce, egg and vanilla; mix well and set aside.

3. In a separate bowl, combine the CSE Pancake & Waffle Mix, protein powder, flaxseed meal, baking soda, baking powder and sea salt. Add the wet ingredients to the dry ingredients and whisk together until just combined.

4. Line a muffin tin with liners. Scoop about ¼ cup of the batter into each muffin cup and top with chocolate chips. Bake for 15-16 minutes. Transfer from the pan to the cooling rack.

Add one of these protein options on the side:
1 muffin + 3 scrambled egg whites
230 calories / 6.5F / 27.5C / 17P

1 muffin + ½ serving CSE Simply Vanilla Protein Powder
230 calories / 6F / 31C / 16P

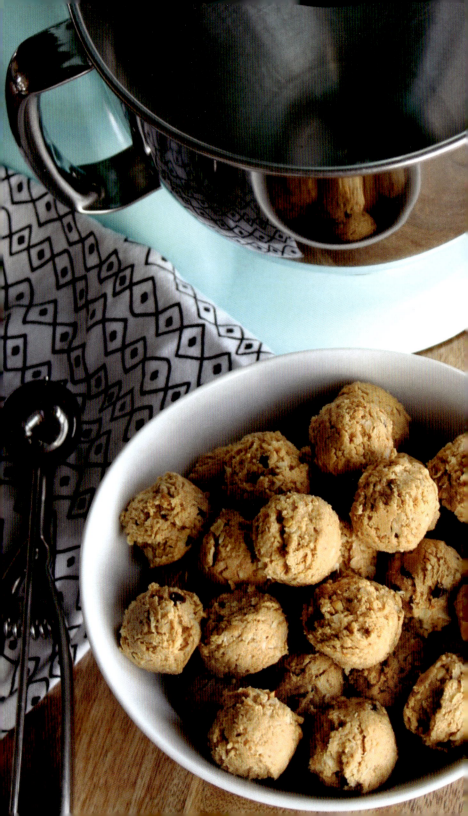

CHOCOLATE CHIP COOKIE DOUGH BITES

Makes 26 bites
95 calories / 5F / 11.5C / 3.5P / per bite

1 cup OffBeat Sweet Classic Peanut Butter
   or natural peanut butter
½ cup raw honey
1 tsp. vanilla extract
1 serving CSE Simply Vanilla Protein Powder
1 ½ cups Oat Flour
Dash of sea salt
30 dark chocolate chips

1. Add all the ingredients to a large bowl and mix until well combined.

2. Using a small cookie scoop, scoop into balls and store in the fridge or freezer. Enjoy!

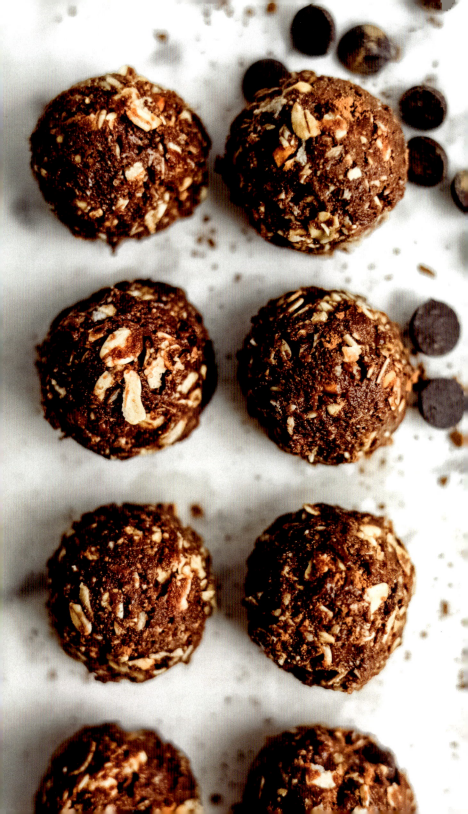

DARK CHOCOLATE PEANUT BUTTER BITES

Makes 26 bites
110 calories / 5.5F / 11.5C / 4P / per bite

---

1 cup OffBeat Sweet Classic Peanut Butter, Buckeye Brownie Butter
   or natural peanut butter
½ cup raw honey
1 serving CSE Brownie Batter or Chocolate Peanut Butter
   Protein Powder
1 ½ cup old-fashioned rolled oats
2 Tbs. cocoa powder
30 extra dark chocolate chips

1. Add all the ingredients to a large bowl and mix until well combined.

2. Using a small cookie scoop, scoop into balls and store in the fridge or freezer. Enjoy!

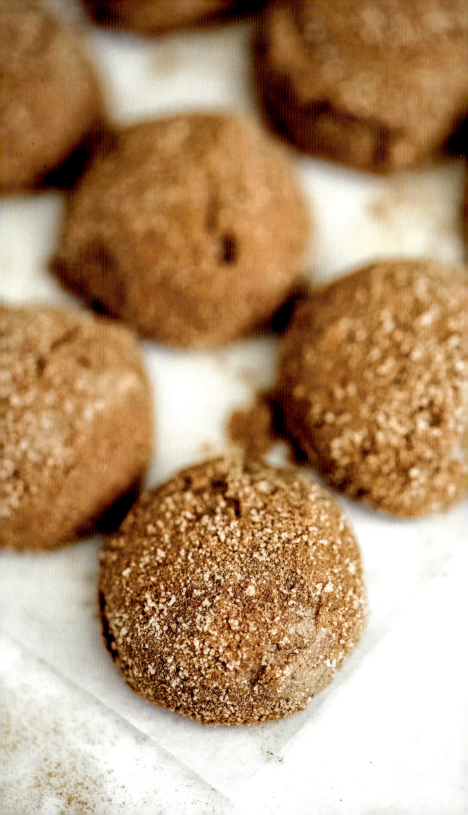

SNICKERDOODLE BITES
Makes 26 bites
100 calories / 5F / 11C / 3.5P / per bite

1 cup OffBeat Cinnamon Bun Butter
  or natural almond butter
½ cup pure maple syrup
2 servings CSE Snickerdoodle or Simply Vanilla Protein Powder
1 ½ cups oat flour
½ tsp. butter extract
½ tsp vanilla extract
Dash of sea salt
Optional Toppings:
1 Tbs. Truvia
½ Tbs. cinnamon

1. Add all the ingredients to a large bowl and mix until well combined.

2. Using a small cookie scoop, scoop into balls and store in the fridge or freezer. Enjoy!

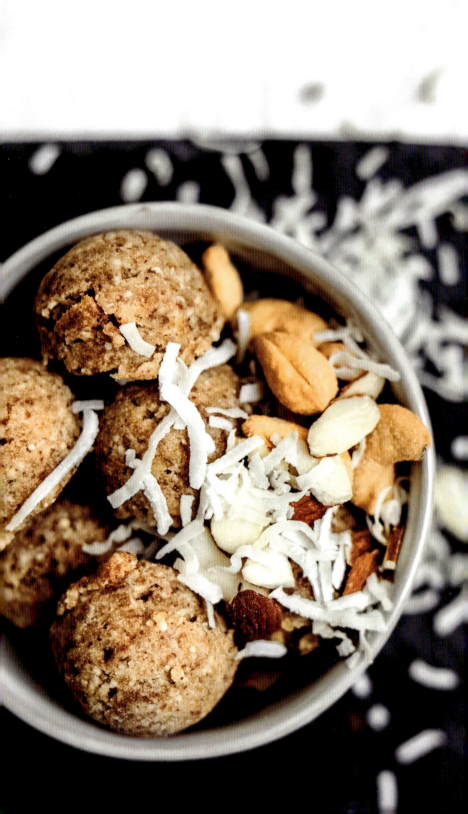

SWEET COCONUTTY ENERGY BITES

Makes 20 bites
100 calories / 6F / 11C / 3P / per bite

½ cup almonds
½ cup cashews
½ cup unsweetened shredded coconut
1 ½ cups pitted dates
1 Tbs. coconut oil
1 serving CSE Simply Vanilla or Coconut Cream Protein Powder
Dash sea salt

1. Add almonds, cashews and coconut to a food processor or high-powered blender. Pulse until nuts are finely chopped. Add dates and coconut oil. Pulse until dates are finely chopped and mixture begins to stick together. Stir in protein powder and sea salt; Mix well.

2. Using a small cookie scoop, scoop into balls and store in the fridge or freezer. Enjoy!

*If too crumbly, add a little bit of almond milk to help form.

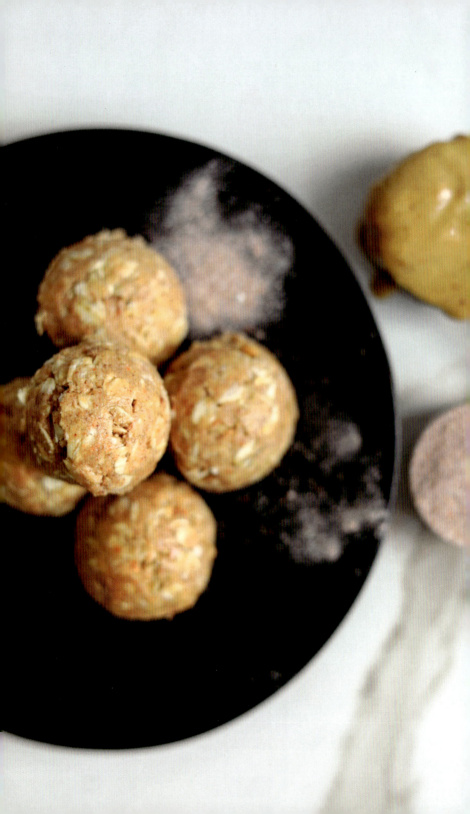

PB&J POWER BITES

Makes 26 bites
65 calories / 3F / 7C / 3P / per bite

1 cup OffBeat Sweet Classic Peanut Butter
   or natural peanut butter
½ cup raw honey
2 servings CSE Simply Vanilla or Strawberry Cheesecake
   Protein Powder
2 servings CSE Super Berry Mix
1 ½ cups old-fashioned rolled oats
Dash vanilla extract
Dash sea salt

1. Add all the ingredients to a large bowl and mix until well combined.

2. Using a small cookie scoop, scoop into balls and store in the fridge or freezer. Enjoy!

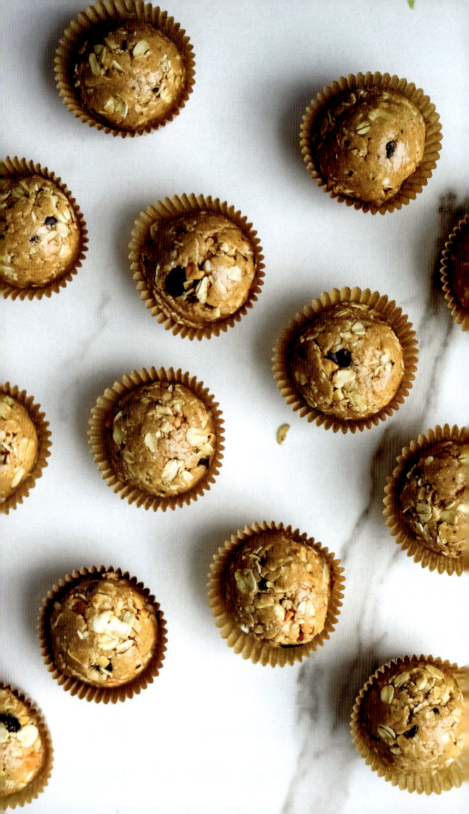

TRIPLE-CHIP BUTTERSCOTCH BITES
Makes 30 servings / 1 per serving
100 calories / 5F / 10.5C / 4P / per serving

---

1 cup OffBeat Sweet Classic Peanut Butter
   or natural peanut butter
½ cup raw honey
½ tsp. vanilla extract
2 servings CSE Simply Vanilla Protein Powder
1 ½ cups old-fashioned rolled oats
Dash of sea salt
1 Tbs. chopped butterscotch chips
1 Tbs. chopped dark chocolate chips
1 Tbs. chopped white chocolate chips

1. Add all the ingredients to a large bowl and mix until well combined.

2. Using a small cookie scoop, scoop into balls and store in the fridge or freezer. Enjoy!

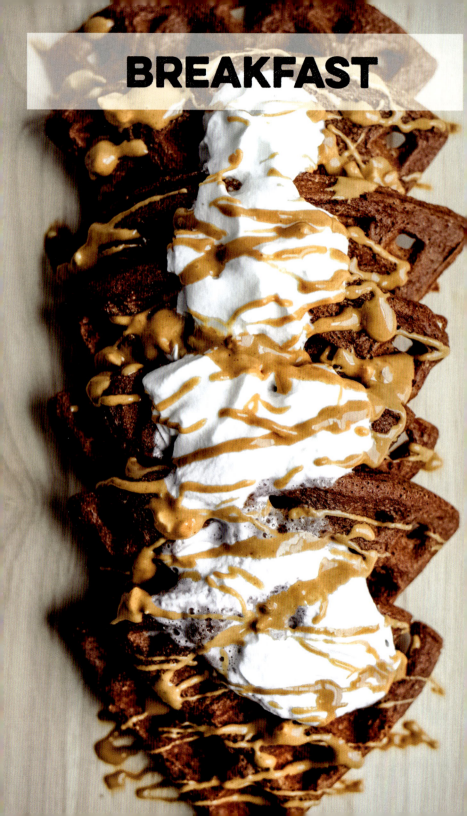

BREAKFAST

I LOVE SLEEP
BECAUSE IT'S
LIKE A TIME
MACHINE TO
BREAKFAST

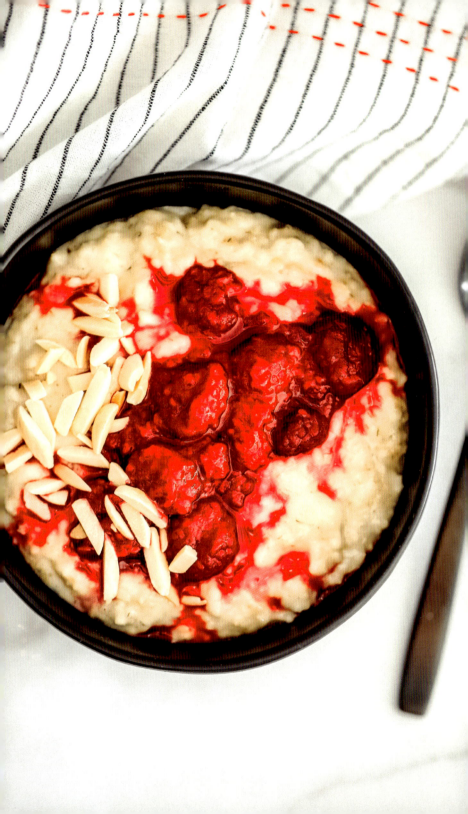

RASPBERRY ALMOND OATS

Makes 1 serving
340 calories / 10.5F / 35C / 26.5P

⅓ cup old-fashioned rolled oats
½ cup water
2 Tbs. liquid egg whites
½ Tbs. OffBeat Salted Caramel Butter
   or natural almond butter
⅛ tsp. almond extract
Vanilla stevia drops, optional
¼ cup nonfat, plain Greek yogurt
½ serving CSE Simply Vanilla Protein Powder
⅓ cup fresh or frozen raspberries
1 Tbs. sliced almonds

1. Mix oats, egg whites and water together in a bowl.

2. Microwave for 1-2 minutes.

3. Stir in the nut butter of choice, almond extract, stevia and Greek yogurt. Add in the protein powder last and mix until well combined.

4. Heat the raspberries in the microwave for 30-60 seconds or in a small saucepan on the stovetop. Cook until melted down and warm. Add to the oatmeal and top with sliced almonds.

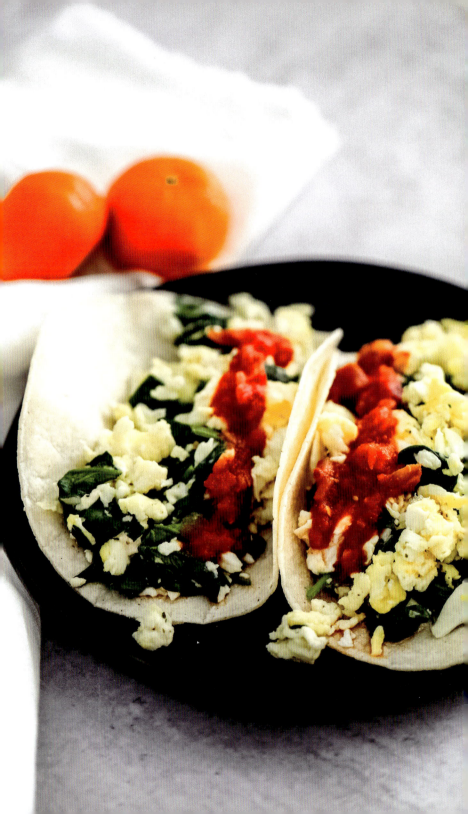

BREAKFAST TACOS

Makes 2 servings
350 calories / 12F / 34C / 26P / per serving

---

3 large eggs
6 egg whites
1 cup chopped spinach
2 light Laughing Cow cheese wedges
4 corn tortillas
2 Tbs. salsa
2 clementine oranges

1. Scramble the eggs and egg whites together with spinach and cheese. Remove from pan.

2. Divide the egg mixture evenly between four tortillas and top each taco with ½ Tbs. salsa. Enjoy two tacos per serving and one orange on the side.

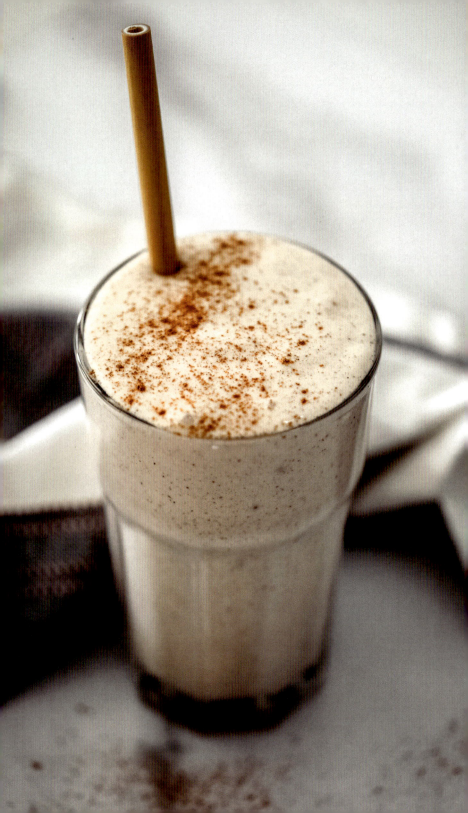

CINNAMON ROLL SHAKE

Makes 1 serving
350 calories / 12F / 34.5C / 26.5P

¾ cup unsweetened almond milk
¼ cup nonfat, plain Greek yogurt
¾ serving CSE Simply Vanilla or Cinnamon Roll Protein Powder
50g frozen banana slices
2 Tbs. old-fashioned rolled oats
1 Tbs. OffBeat Cinnamon Bun Butter
   or 3 Tbs. Neufchâtel cream cheese
1 tsp. coconut sugar
1 tsp. cinnamon
6-8 (120g) ice cubes

1. Add all of the ingredients to a high-powered blender. Blend on high until smooth. Enjoy!

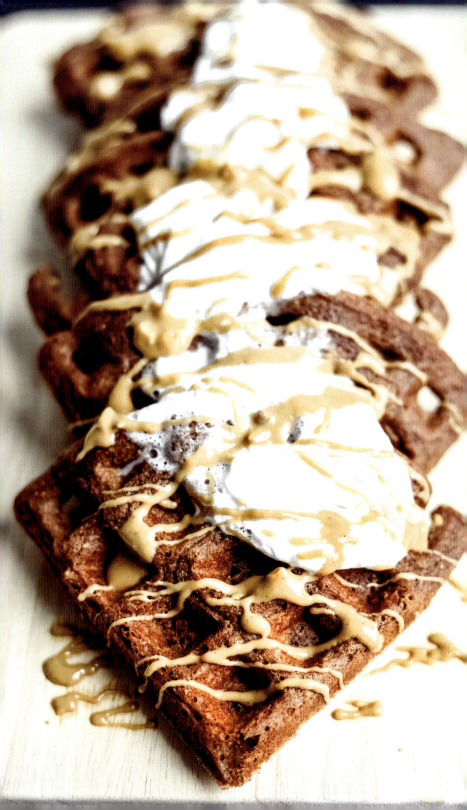

CHOCOLATE WAFFLES

Makes 4 servings
350 calories / 12F / 36C / 25.5P / per serving

1 cup CSE Vanilla Pancake & Waffle Mix
1 serving CSE Brownie Batter Protein Powder
1 Tbs. cocoa powder
1 ¾ cups water
2 large eggs
40g mashed banana

Toppings per serving:
1 Tbs. OffBeat Sweet Classic Peanut Butter, Buckeye Brownie
   Butter or natural peanut butter
2 Tbs. spray whipped cream topping
Zero calorie syrup of choice

1. Preheat waffle iron.

2. In a medium-sized bowl, mix together the CSE Pancake & Waffle Mix, protein powder, cocoa powder, water, eggs, and banana. Stir together until well combined.

3. Spray the waffle iron with cooking spray. Pour the batter into the waffle iron. Repeat with the remaining batter. Weigh the waffles and divide the weight by four to get the amount needed to fill one serving.

3. Top each serving with 1 Tbs. peanut butter, 2 Tbs. whipped cream and syrup. Enjoy!

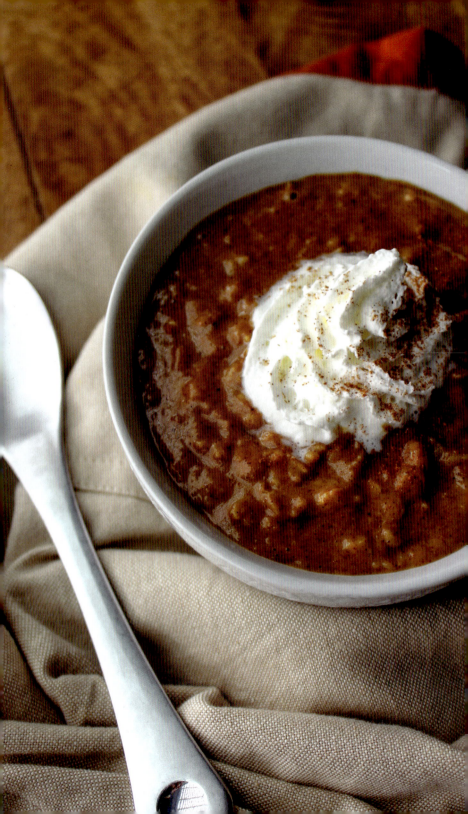

GINGERBREAD COOKIE OATMEAL

Makes 1 serving
340 calories / 11F / 38C / 22P

⅓ cup old-fashioned rolled oats
½ cup water
3 Tbs. liquid egg whites
1 Tbs. OffBeat Gingerbread Cookie Butter
   or natural almond butter
2 tsp. molasses
¼ tsp. ground cinnamon
Dash ground ginger
Dash sea salt
½ serving CSE Simply Vanilla Protein Powder
Topping:
2 Tbs. spray whipped cream topping

1. Mix oats, water and egg whites together in a bowl.

2. Microwave for 1-2 minutes.

3. Stir in the nut butter and molasses. Then add in the spices and protein powder. Top with whipped cream; enjoy warm.

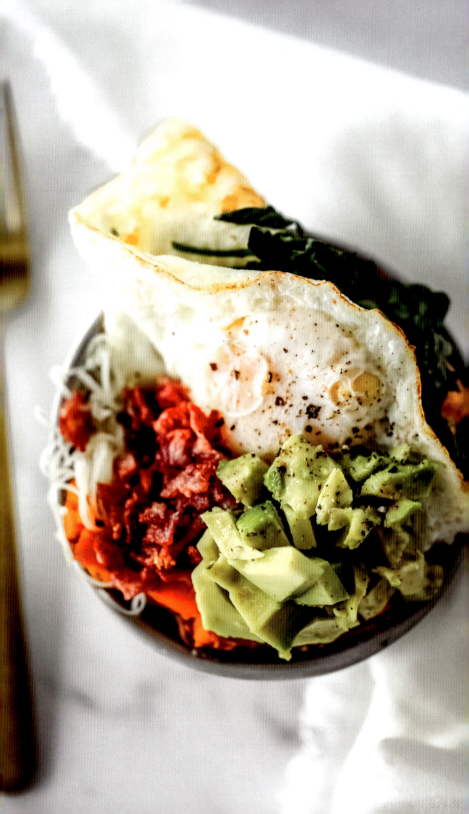

BREAKFAST SWEET POTATO

Makes 1 serving
350 calories / 11.5F / 35C / 26P

150g baked sweet potato
1 slice turkey bacon
1 large egg
2 egg whites
1 cup spinach
1 Tbs. low-fat, shredded mozzarella cheese
25g chopped avocado
Sea salt and pepper, to taste

1. Bake the sweet potato in the oven or microwave according to the directions in the Food Prep Guide.

2. Chop the bacon. Spray a sauté pan and heat to medium/high. Add the bacon and cook until crispy. Remove from the pan. Spray the pan again and add the egg, egg whites and spinach.

3. Place the sweet potato on a plate and mash with a fork. Top with eggs, spinach, cheese, bacon and avocado; salt and pepper to taste. Enjoy warm.

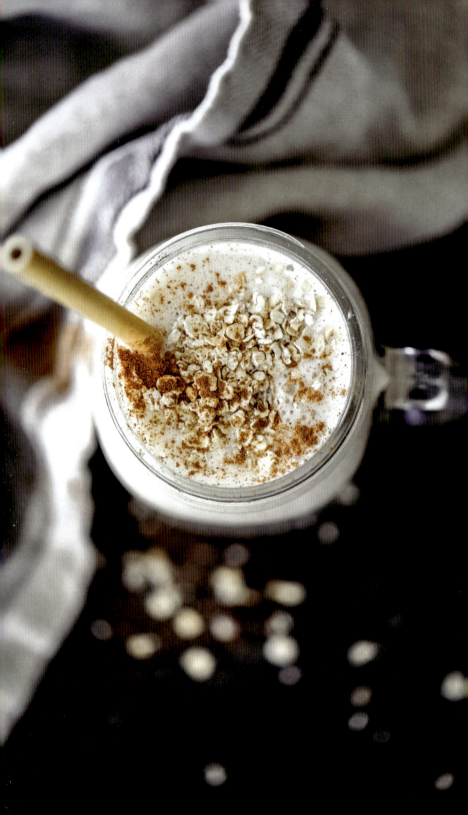

OATMEAL COOKIE SHAKE

Makes 1 serving
350 calories / 12F / 35.5C / 26P

1 cup unsweetened almond milk
½ serving CSE Simply Vanilla Protein Powder
⅓ cup old-fashioned rolled oats
⅓ cup low-fat cottage cheese
10g raisins
2 tsp. OffBeat Cinnamon Bun Butter, Gingerbread Cookie
    Butter or natural almond butter
1 tsp. cinnamon
Dash of sea salt
⅛ tsp. butter extract
6-8 ice cubes

1. Add all of the ingredients to a high-powered blender. Blend on high until smooth.

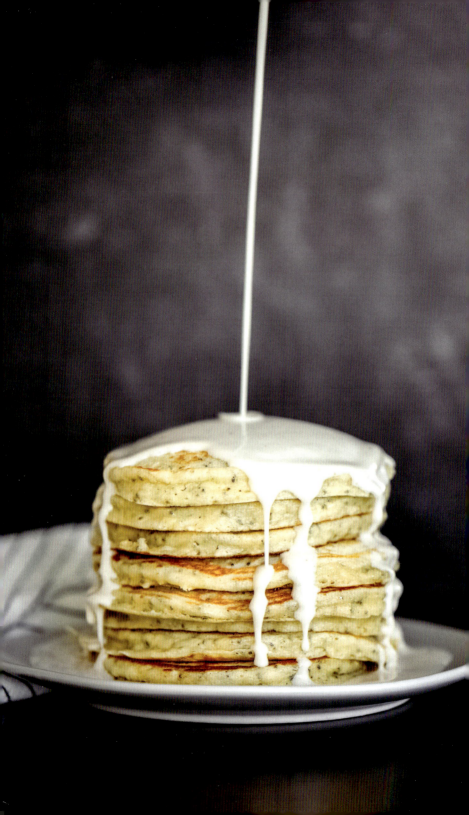

LEMON CHIA PANCAKES

Makes 4 servings
350 calories / 12F / 31C / 28.5P / per serving

---

1 ¾ cups CSE Vanilla Pancake & Waffle Mix
⅓ cup water
1 cup nonfat, plain Greek yogurt
4 large eggs
Vanilla stevia drops, optional
1 ½ Tbs. chia seeds
1 lemon, zest of

Toppings per serving:
1 Tbs. nonfat, plain Greek yogurt
2 Tbs. zero calorie syrup of choice
1 tsp. coconut oil or grass-fed butter

1. Heat a skillet to medium heat.

2. In a large bowl whisk the CSE Pancake & Waffle Mix, water, yogurt, eggs and stevia together. Once combined, stir in the chia seeds and lemon zest.

3. Pour 1/4 cup of the mixture onto the griddle. When small bubbles begin to form on the top, flip the pancakes over. Repeat for the remaining batter. Divide the amount of pancakes made by four to get the amount needed to fill one serving.

4. Stir the Greek yogurt and syrup together in a small bowl. Top each serving with one teaspoon coconut oil or butter, then drizzle the yogurt/syrup mixture over the top.

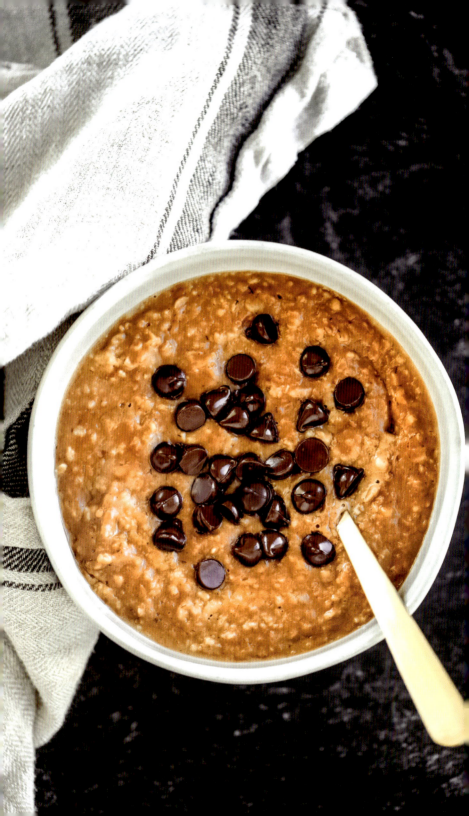

CHOCOLATE PEANUT BUTTER CUP OATMEAL

Makes 1 serving
340 calories / 11F / 32C / 27P

⅓ cup old-fashioned rolled oats
⅔ cup water
3 Tbs. egg whites
2 Tbs. powdered peanut butter
2 tsp. OffBeat Sweet Classic Peanut Butter
  or natural peanut butter
½ serving CSE Chocolate Peanut Butter or Brownie Batter
  Protein Powder
15 extra dark chocolate chips

1. Mix the oats, water, egg whites and powdered peanut butter together in a bowl.

2. Microwave for 1-2 minutes.

3. Stir in the peanut butter and let cool slightly. Stir in the protein powder and top with dark chocolate chips.

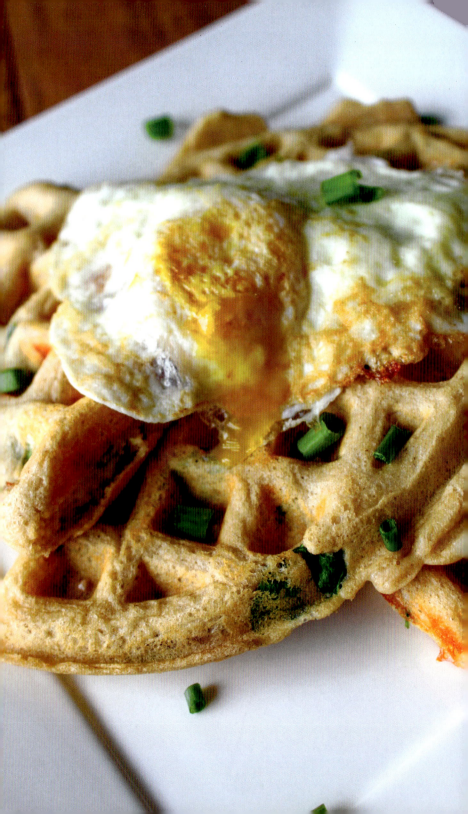

SAVORY STUFFED WAFFLES

Makes 4 servings
335 calories / 10F / 31C / 29.5P / per serving

2 slices turkey bacon
2 cups CSE Vanilla Pancake & Waffle Mix
1 ½ cup water
2 cups chopped spinach
½ cup low-fat, shredded mozzarella cheese
2 Tbs. chopped, fresh chives
4 large eggs
Zero calorie syrup of choice, optional

1. Heat a waffle iron. Chop the bacon and cook in a frying pan over medium-high heat until crispy. Remove from pan.

2. Whisk the CSE Pancake & Waffle Mix and water together in a bowl until well combined. Fold in the bacon, chopped spinach, cheese and chives. Spray the waffle iron with cooking spray and add the batter. Cook until golden brown. Repeat with the remaining batter. Weigh the waffles and divide the weight by four to get the amount needed to fill one serving.

3. While the waffles are cooking, heat the frying pan over medium heat and cook the eggs to your preference. Top each waffle with one egg and a drizzle of syrup, if desired.

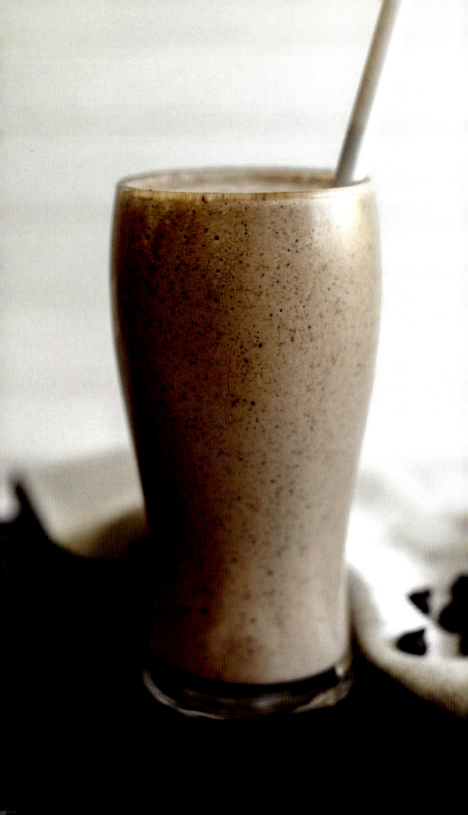

CHOCOLATE CHIP ALMOND MOCHA SHAKE

Makes 1 serving
350 calories / 12F / 33C / 27P

½ cup unsweetened almond milk
½ cup cold brewed coffee or cold brewed Crio Bru
¾ serving (24g) CSE Brownie Batter Protein Powder
100g frozen banana slices
2 Tbs. nonfat, plain Greek yogurt
1 Tbs. OffBeat Almond Mocha Butter
   or natural almond butter
15 extra dark chocolate chips
¼ tsp. almond extract, optional
6-8 (120g) ice cubes

1. Add all of the ingredients to a high-powered blender. Blend on high until smooth.

*For directions and more information on Crio Bru, visit cleansimpleeats.com/blog

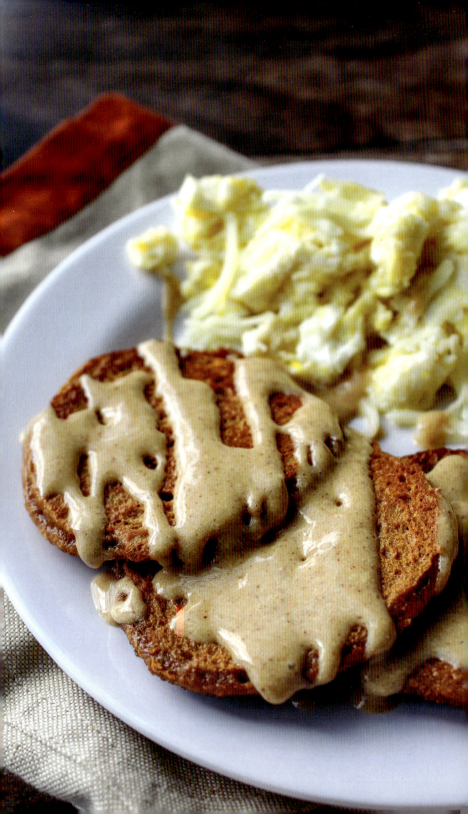

SILVER DOLLAR GINGERBREAD PANCAKES

Makes 4 servings
350 calories / 11F / 34C / 28P / per serving

---

1 cup CSE Vanilla Pancake & Waffle Mix
¼ cup water
3 Tbs. molasses
1 large egg
½ tsp. ground cinnamon
⅛ tsp. ground ginger

Caramel Topping:
½ serving CSE Simply Vanilla Protein Powder
2 Tbs. unsweetened almond milk
1 Tbs. OffBeat Salted Caramel Butter, Gingerbread Cookie
   Butter or natural almond butter
1 Tbs. raw honey

Sides per serving:
1 large egg
2 egg whites
1 Tbs. low-fat, shredded mozzarella cheese

1. Heat a griddle over medium heat.

2. Whisk together the CSE Pancake & Waffle Mix, water, molasses,
egg and spices. Drop by the tablespoon onto the griddle, making
mini pancakes. Divide the total number of pancakes by four to get
the amount needed to fill one serving.

3. Whisk the topping ingredients together in a small bowl. Top
each serving of pancakes with ¼ of the caramel topping.

4. Cook the eggs to your liking and serve on the side.

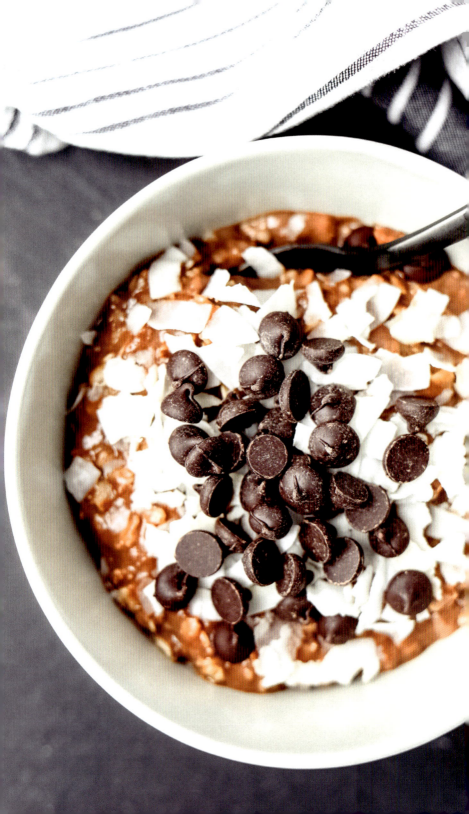

ALMOND JOY OATMEAL

Makes 1 servings
350 calories / 13F / 32C / 26P / per serving

⅓ cup old-fashioned rolled oats
½ cup water
3 Tbs. egg whites
½ Tbs. OffBeat Midnight Almond Coconut Butter
   or natural almond butter
¾ serving (24g) CSE Brownie Batter Protein Powder
5g unsweetened coconut flakes
10g dark chocolate chips

1. Place the oats, water and egg whites in a microwave-safe bowl. Whisk until the egg whites are well combined.

2. Microwave for 1-2 minutes.

3. Stir in the nut butter and then let cool slightly. Stir in the protein powder and top with the coconut flakes and chocolate chips.

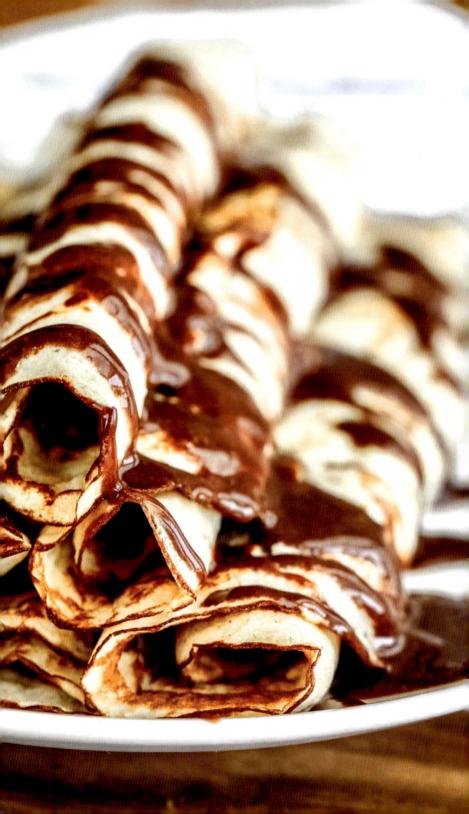

CHOCOLATE GLAZED BANANA CREPES

Makes 4 servings
350 calories / 12.5F / 33C / 26P / per serving

8 (1 cup) egg whites
120g bananas
1 cup CSE Vanilla Pancake & Waffle Mix
1 cup fat-free milk
Pinch of sea salt
1 tsp. Stevia in the Raw, optional
Chocolate Glaze:
2 Tbs. OffBeat Midnight Almond Coconut Butter, Sweet Classic
   Peanut Butter or natural peanut butter
2 Tbs. melted coconut oil
1 serving CSE Brownie Batter Protein Powder
1 Tbs. cocoa powder
1 Tbs. raw honey
¼ cup unsweetened almond milk

1. Heat a frying pan over medium heat. Add the egg whites, banana, CSE Pancake & Waffle Mix, milk, sea salt and stevia together in a high-powered blender. Blend on low for 30 seconds, scrape down the sides and blend for another 30 seconds.

2. Spray the pan with cooking spray and pour ¼ cup of the batter into the pan. Swirl the batter around the sides to make a thin crepe. Once the edges start to peel away from the pan, carefully flip the crepe. Cook for one more minute and then transfer to a plate. Repeat with the rest of the batter. It should make about 12 crepes.

3. Whisk together all of the chocolate glaze ingredients. Weigh the glaze and divide the weight by four to get the amount needed to fill one serving.

4. Roll the banana crepes up and drizzle the chocolate glaze over the top. Enjoy warm.

ENTREES

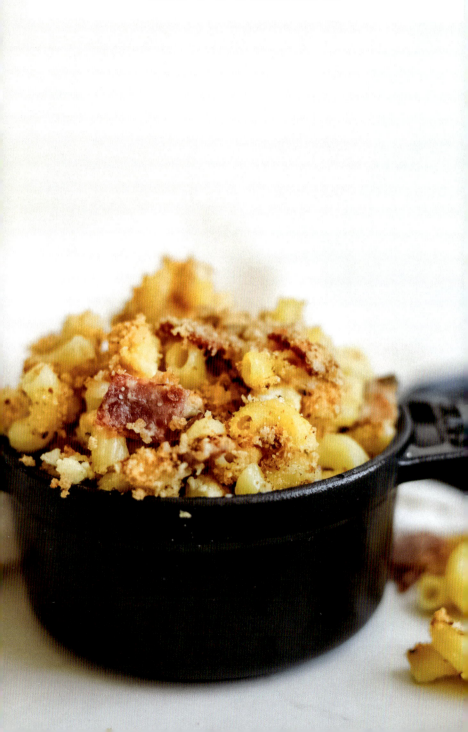

FIRST WE EAT... THEN WE DO EVERYTHING ELSE

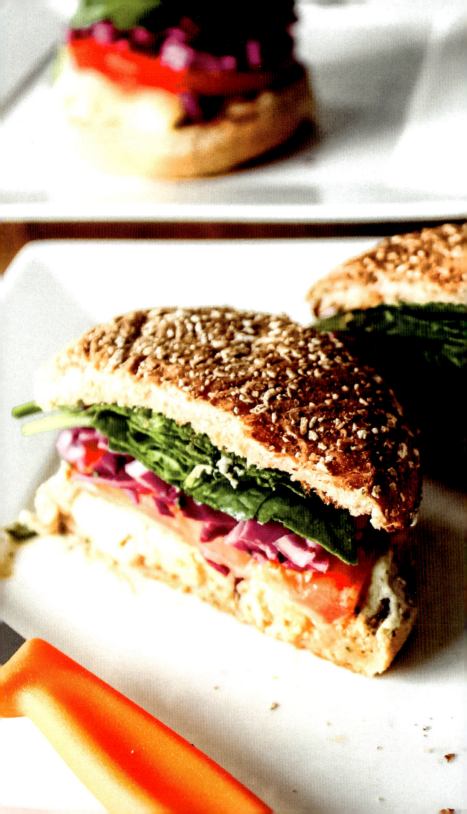

BUFFALO CHICKEN & PESTO SANDWICH

Makes 2 servings
345 calories / 13F / 32C / 25P / per serving

3 oz. cooked chicken breast (4 oz. raw)
2 tsp. Frank's hot sauce
¼ tsp. dried basil
Sea salt and pepper, to taste
2 slices Pepper Jack cheese
1 Tbs. pesto sauce
2 Tbs. nonfat, plain Greek yogurt
2 whole wheat hamburger buns (140 cals each)
1 sliced vine tomato
½ cup spinach
½ cup sliced red cabbage

1. Coat the raw chicken in hot sauce and dried basil. Place in a pan over medium heat, then sprinkle with sea salt and pepper. Cover and cook for three minutes per side or until cooked through. Remove from the heat and separate into two equal portions. Top each portion with one slice of cheese.

2. Stir the pesto sauce and yogurt together in a bowl.

3. Toast the buns then spread ½ of the pesto cream sauce on the bottom of each bun. Add ½ of the chicken, ¼ cup of the cabbage, ¼ cup of the spinach and two tomato slices to each sandwich. Top with the other half of the bun.

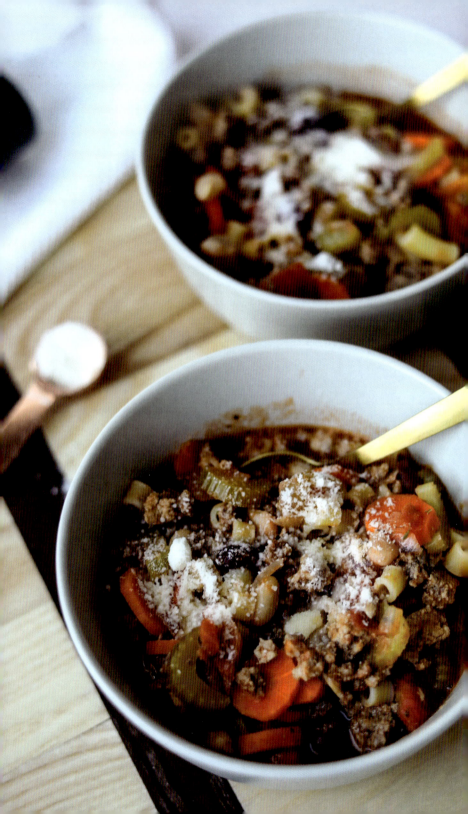

PASTA E FAGIOLI
Makes 4 servings
355 calories / 12F / 36C / 25P / per serving

---

12 oz. lean ground beef
½ cup diced yellow onion
1 tsp. minced garlic
~~2 chopped celery sticks~~
2 sliced, medium-sized carrots
2 cups canned diced tomatoes
½ cup red kidney beans, drained
½ cup great northern beans, drained
1 cup tomato sauce
½ cup vegetable broth
2 tsp. white wine vinegar
½ tsp. dried basil
½ tsp. dried oregano
½ tsp. sea salt
¼ tsp. dried thyme
¼ tsp. ground black pepper
2 oz. uncooked ditalini or macaroni pasta

good!

Topping per serving:
1 tsp. grated Parmesan cheese

1. Brown the ground beef in a large pot over medium heat. Add the onions, garlic, celery and carrots. Sauté for about 10 minutes. Add the remaining ingredients, except for the pasta, and simmer for 30 minutes.

2. Cook the pasta al dente according to the directions on the package; drain.

3. Add the pasta to the pot of soup and then simmer for five minutes. Weigh the entire soup and divide the weight by four to get the amount needed to fill one serving. Serve warm topped with Parmesan cheese.

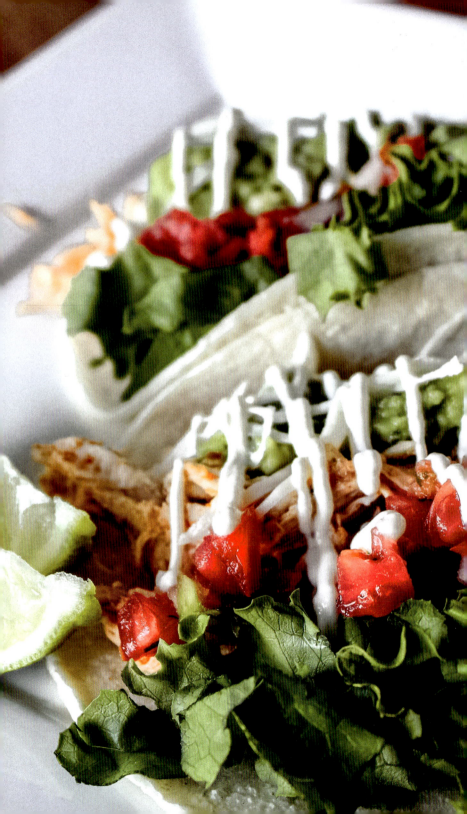

ROTISSERIE CHICKEN TACOS

Makes 4 servings
345 calories / 11F / 36C / 25P / per serving

---

10 oz. shredded rotisserie chicken breast
1-2 Tbs. taco seasoning
8 corn tortillas
4 Tbs. low-fat, shredded mozzarella cheese
4 clementine oranges
Toppings per serving:
½ cup shredded lettuce
1 Tbs. guacamole
2 Tbs. Pico de Gallo
1 Tbs. Cashew Sour Cream
½ lime, juice of
Cilantro, for garnish

1. Prepare the Cashew Sour Cream. Recipe in the Food Prep Guide.

2. Preheat the oven to HI broil. Shred the chicken into a bowl and stir in the taco seasoning. Lay the tortillas out on a pan and fill each tortilla with 1.25 ounces shredded chicken and a ½ tablespoon shredded mozzarella cheese.

3. Place in the oven and broil for three minutes or until the cheese is melted.

4. Remove from oven and add all the toppings to each taco. Two tacos per serving. Enjoy one clementine on the side.

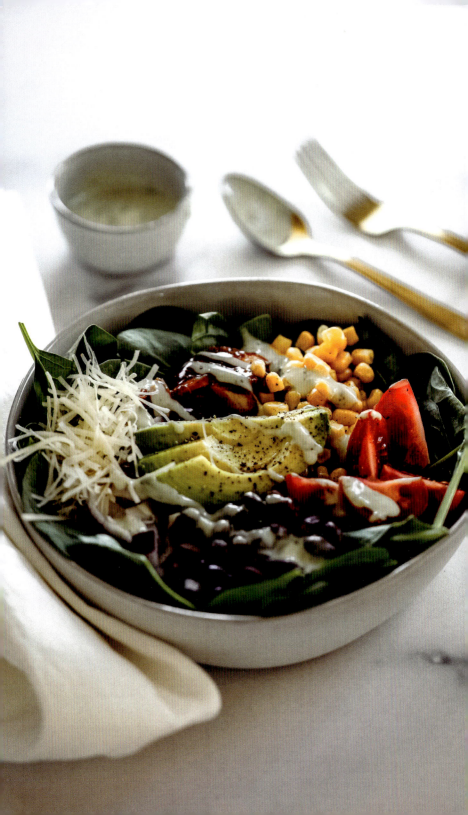

BBQ CHICKEN CHOPPED SALAD

Makes 4 servings
345 calories / 12F / 33C / 24P / per serving

---

8 oz. cooked chicken breast (10.6 oz. raw)
½ cup Stubbs BBQ Sauce
8 cups chopped spinach
1 cup black beans, drained and rinsed
1 cup frozen corn, thawed
2 diced vine tomatoes
½ cup diced red onion
Toppings per serving:
30 grams chopped avocado
2 Tbs. Bolthouse Farms Cilantro Avocado Dressing
1 Tbs. grated Parmesan cheese

1. Cook or grill the chicken according to the directions in the Food Prep Guide.

2. Cube or shred the chicken and mix together with the BBQ sauce.

3. For one serving, layer two cups of chopped spinach, ¼ of the BBQ chicken mixture, ¼ cup of the black beans, ¼ cup of the corn, ½ of a diced tomato, two tablespoons diced red onion, 30g avocado, two tablespoons of the dressing and one tablespoon Parmesan cheese.

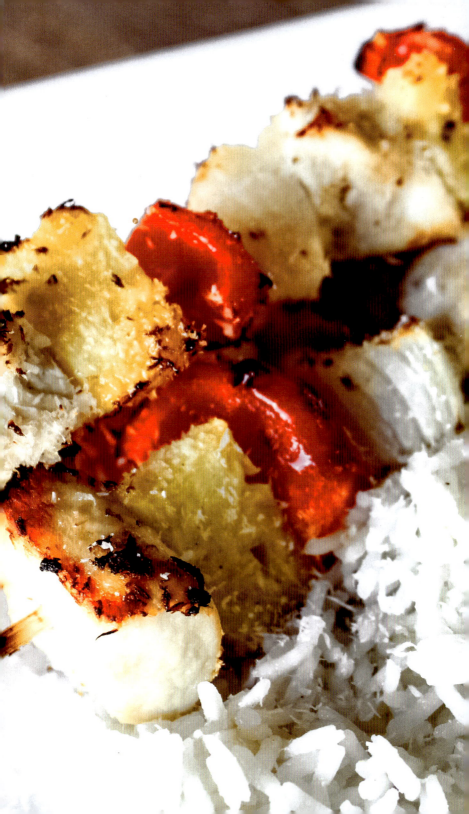

ALOHA CHICKEN KABOBS

Makes 4 servings
350 calories / 11F / 36C / 27P / per serving

Wooden skewer sticks
6 Tbs. uncooked white jasmine rice
¾ cup full-fat, canned coconut milk
14 oz. raw chicken breast (10.5 oz. cooked)
1 cup chopped red bell peppers
1 cup chopped yellow sweet onions
4 oz. cubed fresh pineapple
1 Tbs. coconut aminos or soy sauce
½ Tbs. raw honey
1 tsp. olive oil
1 tsp. rice vinegar
½ tsp. fresh, minced garlic
½ tsp. ground ginger
Sea salt and pepper, to taste
2 Tbs. unsweetened shredded coconut

1. Soak the skewer sticks for an hour before cooking.

2. Heat oven to HI broil.

3. Cook the rice according to directions on package, using coconut milk for the liquid instead of water. Stir in a pinch of sea salt. Weigh or measure the rice and divide by four to get the amount needed to fill one serving.

4. Cube the chicken. Measure out 3.5 ounces raw, cubed chicken, ¼ cup peppers, ¼ cup onions and 1 ounce pineapple. Skewer in a pattern then place onto a greased broiler pan; set aside.

5. Combine the coconut aminos, honey, olive oil, rice vinegar, minced garlic and ground ginger together in a small bowl. Baste the skewers with the mixture and then sprinkle with sea salt and pepper.

6. Broil for 10-15 minutes, flipping halfway. Sprinkle the shredded coconut over the top. Enjoy warm over coconut rice.

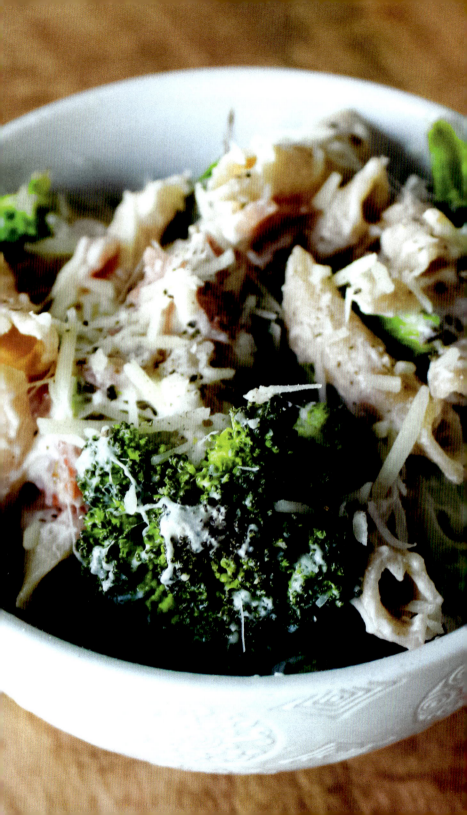

CHEESY BROCCOLI & BACON PENNE

Makes 4 servings
345 calories / 12F / 35C / 24P / per serving

---

4 cups broccoli
4 oz. uncooked, whole-wheat penne pasta
Pinch of sea salt
1 Tbs. olive oil
6 slices turkey bacon, chopped
¼ cup fresh, minced yellow onion
1 tsp. fresh, minced garlic
¼ cup unsweetened almond milk
4 light Laughing Cow cheese wedges
½ cup low-fat, shredded mozzarella cheese
¼ cup grated Parmesan cheese

1. Roast broccoli according to directions in the Food Prep Guide.

2. Cook the pasta with sea salt according to directions on package; drain. Remove the pot from the heat and add pasta back to the pot with the olive oil.

3. Heat a frying pan over medium-high heat. Spray with cooking spray and add the chopped bacon. Cook until crispy, then remove from pan. Turn the heat down to medium/low. Add the onions and garlic; sauté until tender. Add the almond milk and cheese wedges; stir until cheese is completely melted.

4. Add the cheese mixture, bacon and broccoli to the pasta. Stir until well combined. Stir in the shredded mozzarella and Parmesan cheeses. Weigh the entire recipe and divide the weight by four to get the amount needed to fill one serving. Enjoy warm. Add sea salt and pepper, to taste.

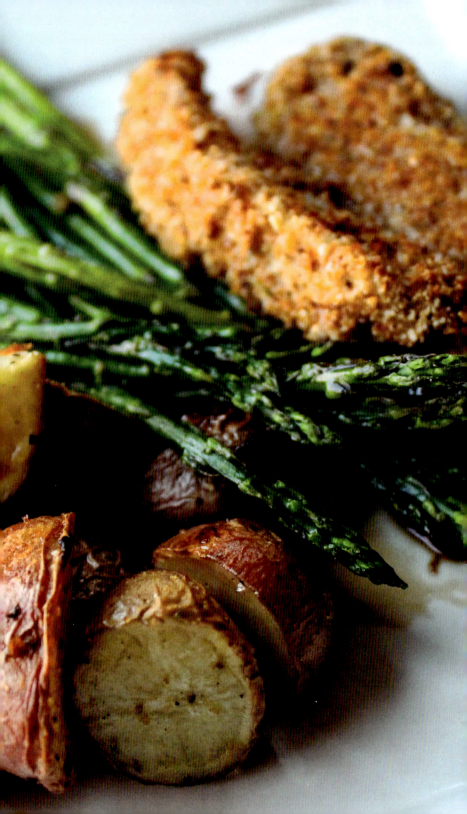

PARMESAN CHICKEN

Makes 4 servings
350 calories / 12F / 36C / 25P / per serving

1 slice Ezekiel Bread or Harper's Bran Bread
1 oz. almonds
2 Tbs. grated Parmesan cheese
¼ tsp. granulated garlic
¼ tsp. dried thyme
½ tsp. sea salt
Dash of ground black pepper
18 oz. baby red potatoes
1 Tbs. olive oil
2 tsp. fresh, minced garlic
9 oz. raw chicken tenderloins (6.75 oz. cooked)
1 egg white
48 asparagus spears
4 tsp. balsamic glaze

1. Toast the bread in the toaster until lightly browned. Place the toast into a blender with the almonds, Parmesan cheese, granulated garlic, thyme, sea salt and pepper. Pulse until broken up into crumbs; set aside.

2. Heat the oven to 400 degrees. Halve the potatoes and place in a large Ziploc bag. Add the olive oil, minced garlic and a dash of sea salt and black pepper to the bag. Massage until well coated. Pour out onto a baking sheet lined with parchment paper. Bake for 20 minutes; flip and bake an additioinal 20 minutes.

3. Dip the chicken tenderloins in the egg whites and then dip into the bread crumb mixture. Place on a baking sheet lined with parchment paper. Bake at 400 degrees for eight minutes. Flip the chicken over and add the asparagus to the pan. Spray the tops with cooking spray and sprinkle with sea salt. Bake the chicken and aparagus together for an additional eight minutes. Drizzle the balsamic glaze over the asparagus. Divide everything evenly into four servings.

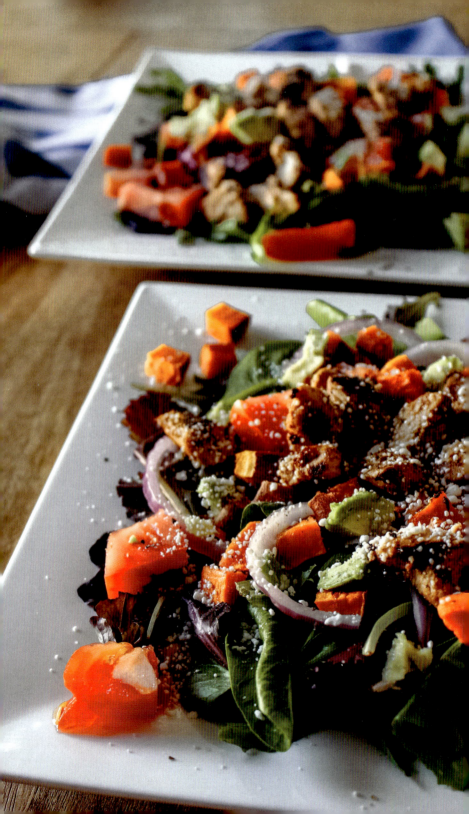

BALSAMIC CHICKEN CHOPPED SALAD

Makes 4 servings
345 calories / 12F / 32C / 27P / per serving

12 oz. raw sweet potatoes
12 oz. raw chicken breast (8 oz. cooked)
¼ cup balsamic vinegar
2 Tbs. olive oil
1 Tbs. water
2 tsp. raw honey
1 tsp. Italian seasoning
1 tsp. fresh, minced garlic
Dash of sea salt
8 cups spring salad mix
2 vine tomatoes, chopped
½ cup red onion, chopped
60g avocado, chopped
4 Tbs. feta cheese crumbles
Sea salt and pepper, to taste

1. Cube and roast sweet potatoes according to directions in the Food Prep Guide.

2. Cube the chicken; set aside. Whisk balsamic vinegar, olive oil, water, honey, Italian seasoning, garlic and sea salt together in a small bowl. Add two tablespoons of the marinade to a bag with the cubed chicken and let sit for 10 minutes. Weigh the remaining marinade and divide the weight by four to get the amount needed to fill one serving of dressing for the salad.

3. Heat a skillet over medium-high heat. Add the chicken and cook until all sides are golden and the chicken is cooked through.

4. For one serving lay 2 cups spring mix out on a plate and then layer with ¼ of the cooked chicken, ¼ of the roasted sweet potatoes, chopped tomato, red onion, 15g avocado, one tablespoon feta cheese and ¼ of the remaining dressing/marinade. Season with salt and pepper to taste.

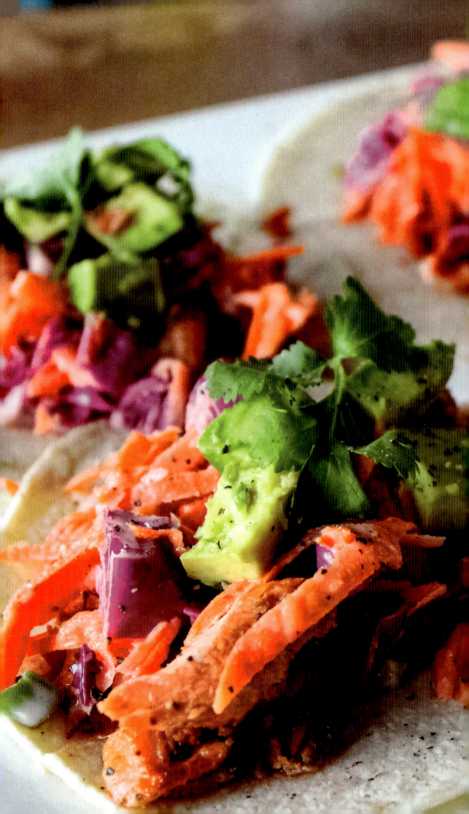

CITRUS SALMON TACOS

Makes 4 servings
350 calories / 13F / 36C / 23P / per serving

---

12 oz. wild caught salmon
½ cup Stubb's Citrus & Onion Marinade
2 cups shredded cabbage
5 oz. grated carrots
2 Tbs. sliced green onions
4 Tbs. nonfat, plain Greek yogurt
1 lime, juice of
Stevia in the Raw, to taste
8 corn tortillas
Sea salt and pepper, to taste
120g chopped avocado
4 Tbs. finely grated Parmesan cheese
Cilantro, for garnish

1. Place the salmon in a Ziploc bag with the marinade. Let marinate 2+ hours or overnight.

2. Spray a frying pan with cooking spray. Remove the salmon from the marinade and pan-fry over medium heat. Cook for five minutes per side or until the salmon begins to flake.

3. In a bowl, combine the cabbage, carrots, green onions, yogurt, lime juice and stevia. Stir until well combined.

4. Assemble tacos by evenly distributing the salmon and cabbage slaw between the tortillas. Season each taco with salt and pepper to taste. Top each taco with 15g of the avocado, ½ tablespoon of the grated Parmesan cheese and a pinch of cilantro. Two tacos per serving.

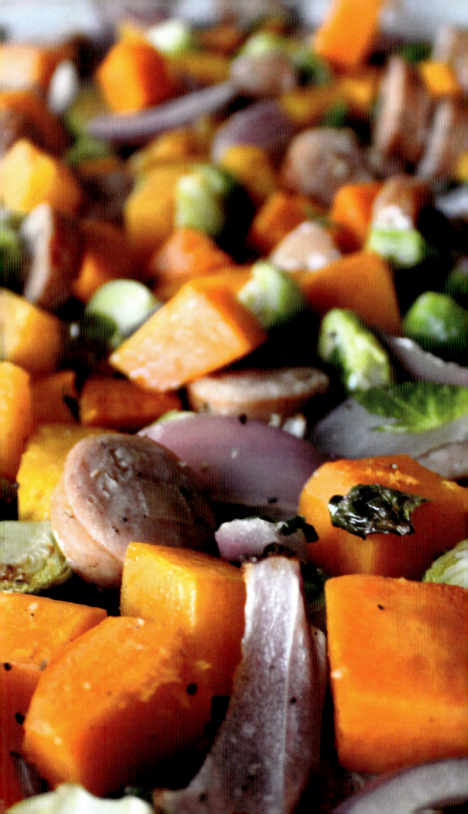

ROASTED WINTER SQUASH & SAUSAGE
Makes 4 servings
330 calories / 12F / 33C / 23P / per serving

5 large chicken sausage links
24 oz. butternut squash, peeled
4 cups Brussels sprouts
1 red onion
2 cloves garlic
1 Tbs. fresh rosemary, chopped (1 tsp. dried)
1 Tbs. fresh sage, chopped (1 tsp. dried)
Dash sea salt
Dash ground pepper

1. Preheat oven to 425 degrees.

2. Slice the chicken sausage. Cube the butternut squash. Trim the Brussels sprouts and slice them in half. Cut the red onion in half and then slice thick. Mince the garlic cloves.

3. Combine the sausage and veggies together in a large bowl with the spices and seasonings. Spread out onto a baking sheet lined with parchment paper. Spray tops with cooking spray and roast for 20 minutes. Flip and roast for another 15-20 minutes or until veggies are lightly browned and tender. Weigh the entire recipe and divide the weight by four to get the amount needed to fill one serving. Enjoy warm.

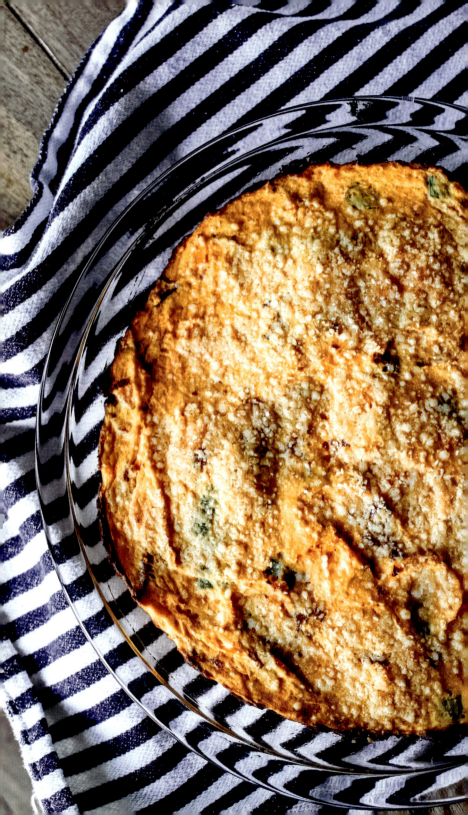

SWEET POTATO PIE

Makes 4 servings
340 calories / 11F / 36C / 24P / per serving

24 oz. raw sweet potatoes
8 slices turkey bacon
4 large eggs
½ cup grated Parmesan cheese
¼ cup sliced green onions
2 tsp. minced garlic
Dash of ground cumin
Dash of sea salt

1. Cook sweet potatoes whole, according to the directions in the Food Prep Guide.

2. Preheat oven to 350 degrees.

3. Chop bacon and cook in a small frying pan over medium heat until crispy.

4. Place the cooked sweet potatoes, bacon, eggs, six tablespoons grated Parmesan cheese, green onions, garlic, cumin and sea salt together in a bowl. Beat with a hand mixer until smooth.

5. Place mixture into a greased pie round or an 8x8 baking dish. Sprinkle with the remaining two tablespoons of Parmesan cheese. Bake for 30-35 minutes or until edges begin to brown. Slice into four equal portions. Enjoy warm.

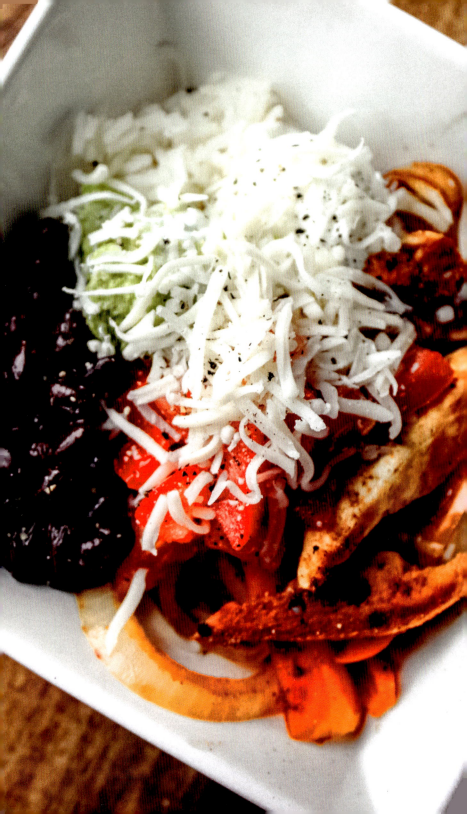

MEXICAN FAJITA BOWL

Makes 4 servings
345 calories / 10F / 36C / 27P / per serving

---

1 cup cooked (⅓ cup uncooked) white jasmine rice
10 oz. raw chicken breast (7.5 oz. cooked)
1 Tbs. taco seasoning
1 red bell pepper, thinly sliced
1 yellow onion, thinly sliced
1 cup black beans, drained and rinsed

Toppings per serving:
2 oz. guacamole
2 Tbs. salsa
2 Tbs. low-fat, shredded mozzarella cheese
1 Tbs. nonfat, plain Greek yogurt
½ lime, juice of

1. Cook the rice according to the directions on the package.

2. Slice chicken thin and sprinkle with taco seasoning. Spray a skillet and add the chicken; cook thoroughly. Add the thinly sliced peppers and onions; sauté until tender.

3. In a bowl layer ¼ of the cooked rice, ¼ of the cooked chicken, ¼ of the onions and peppers, ¼ cup black beans and all the toppings. Enjoy warm.

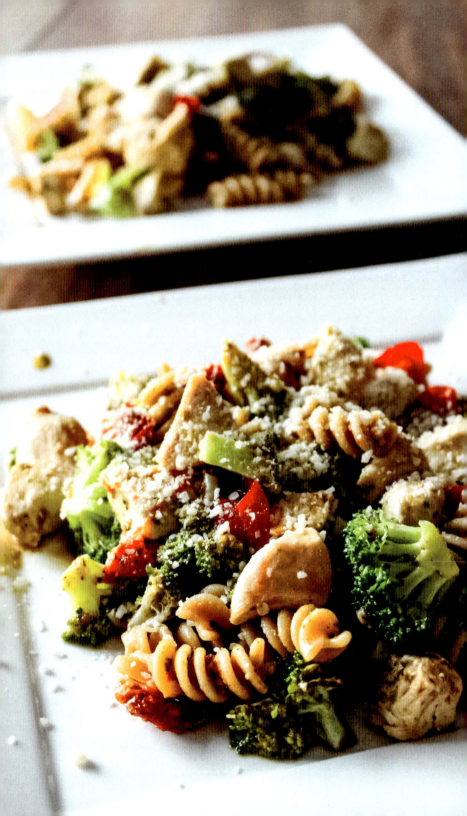

PESTO TOMATO & BROCCOLI FUSILLI
Makes 4 servings
345 calories / 11F / 33C / 28P / per serving

8 oz. cooked chicken breast (10.6 oz. raw)
5 oz. uncooked whole grain fusilli pasta
2 Tbs. pasta water
4 Tbs. pesto sauce
1 cup cherry tomatoes
4 cups chopped broccoli
4 Tbs. shredded Parmesan cheese
Sea salt and pepper, to taste
Red pepper flakes, to taste

1. Cook or grill chicken according to the directions in the Food Prep Guide.

2. Cook pasta according to the directions on the package. Drain pasta water into a bowl and reserve for later use.

3. Heat a skillet to medium heat. Add one tablespoon pesto sauce, cherry tomatoes and broccoli florets. Sauté for three minutes. Turn skillet to low to keep warm.

4. Add pasta, pasta water, cooked chicken, three tablespoons pesto sauce, sea salt and pepper and red pepper flakes to the skillet. Let flavors marinate together for about three minutes, stirring constantly. Weigh the entire recipe and divide the weight by four to get the amount needed to fill one serving. Serve each portion hot topped with one tablespoon of Parmesan cheese.

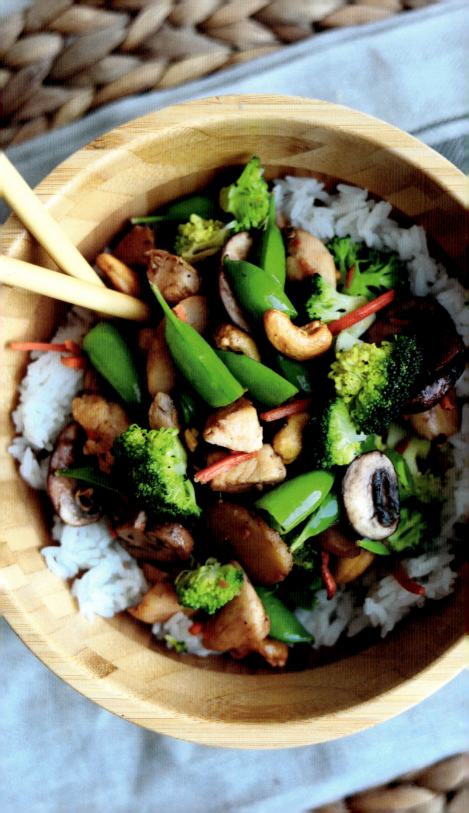

CHICKEN STIR-FRY
Makes 4 servings
330 calories / 11F / 30C / 27P / per serving

1 ⅓ cups cooked (½ cup uncooked) white or brown jasmine rice
14 oz. raw chicken breast (10.5 oz. cooked)
Sea salt and pepper, to taste
2 Tbs. coconut oil
4 Tbs. coconut aminos or soy sauce, divided
1 tsp. fresh, minced garlic
1 cup matchstick carrots
1 cup sugar snap peas, halved
1 cup sliced mushrooms
1 cup chopped broccoli
1 cup water chestnuts
4 Tbs. chopped cashews
Green onions, sliced for garnish

1. Cook rice according to the directions on the package.

2. Heat a skillet to medium heat and spray with cooking spray. Cube chicken and add it to the skillet; sprinkle with sea salt and pepper. Flip the chicken over every three minutes until the chicken is golden on the edges and cooked through. Remove from skillet and set aside.

3. Add the coconut oil, two tablespoons of coconut aminos and garlic to the skillet. Once the oil is melted, add the carrots, pea pods, mushrooms, broccoli and water chestnuts. Sauté about 10 minutes or until the veggies are tender. Add a little sea salt and pepper to taste.

4. Add the cooked chicken and chopped cashews to the skillet and stir together with the veggies. Weigh the entire recipe and divide the weight by four to get the amount needed to fill one serving. Serve each portion over ⅓ cup cooked rice. Top with remaining coconut aminos and sliced green onions.

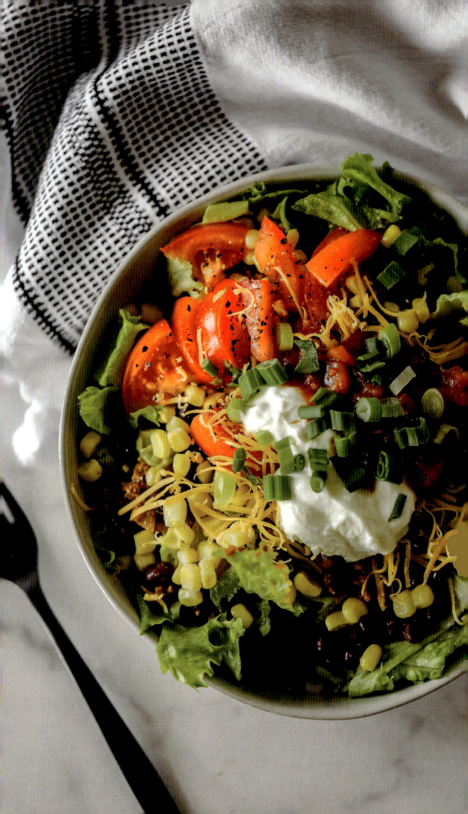

TACO SALAD

Makes 4 servings
350 calories / 13F / 33C / 25P / per serving

---

10 oz. raw lean ground beef
½ cup diced yellow onion
2 Tbs. taco seasoning
8 cups green leaf lettuce
1 cup black beans, rinsed and drained
1 cup frozen corn, thawed
1 cup fresh, diced vine tomatoes
4 Tbs. low-fat, shredded Mexican-style cheese
½ cup nonfat, plain Greek yogurt
½ cup salsa
Green onions, sliced

1. Brown ground beef and onions together in a frying pan over medium/high heat. Add taco seasoning and stir until well coated. Remove from heat. Weigh the meat mixture and divide the weight by four to get the amount needed to fill one serving.

2. Assemble each salad by piling up 2 cups of lettuce, ¼ of the meat mixture, ¼ cup black beans, ¼ cup corn, ¼ cup tomatoes, one tablespoon cheese, two tablespoons plain Greek yogurt and two tablespoons salsa. Garnish with green onions.

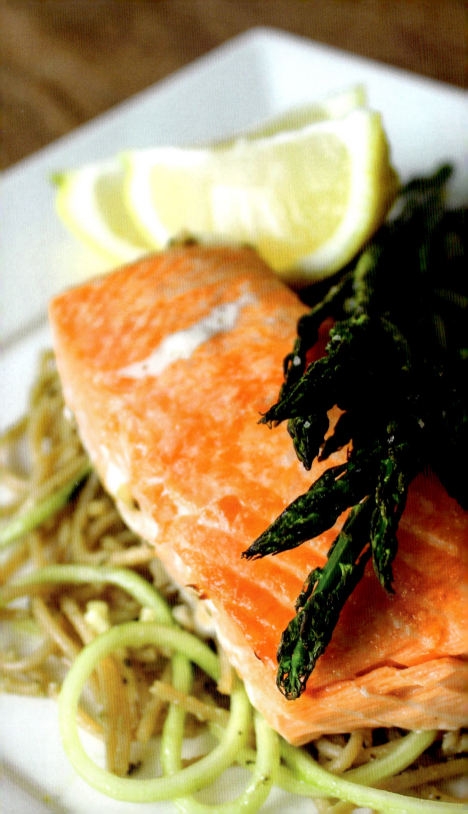

SALMON & GREENS SPAGHETTI

Makes 4 servings
335 calories / 11F / 33C / 26P / per serving

---

12 oz. wild caught salmon
Sea salt and pepper, to taste
24 asparagus spears
5 oz. uncooked, whole-wheat spaghetti
¼ cup pesto sauce
2 cups spiralized zucchini squash
1 lemon, juice of

1. Preheat oven to 450 degrees.

2. Cut the salmon into four, three ounce portions. Season with sea salt and pepper. Place skin-side down on a baking sheet lined with parchment paper. Place asparagus on the same baking sheet. Spray the tops with cooking spray and sprinkle with sea salt. Bake asparagus for 8 minutes. Bake the salmon for 12-15 minutes.

3. Cook the spaghetti according to the directions on the package; drain. Add the spaghetti back to the pot with the pesto sauce. Toss until well coated.

4. Spiralize the zucchini squash. Spray a large frying pan or wok with cooking spray and add then zucchini noodles. Cook over medium-high heat for 3-5 minutes until zucchini is crisp-tender.

5. Weigh the pasta and divide the weight by four to get the amount needed to fill one serving. Add ½ cup cooked zuchinni noodles to each plate then top with pesto pasta, roasted salmon and six asparagus spears. Squeeze lemon juice up over the top.

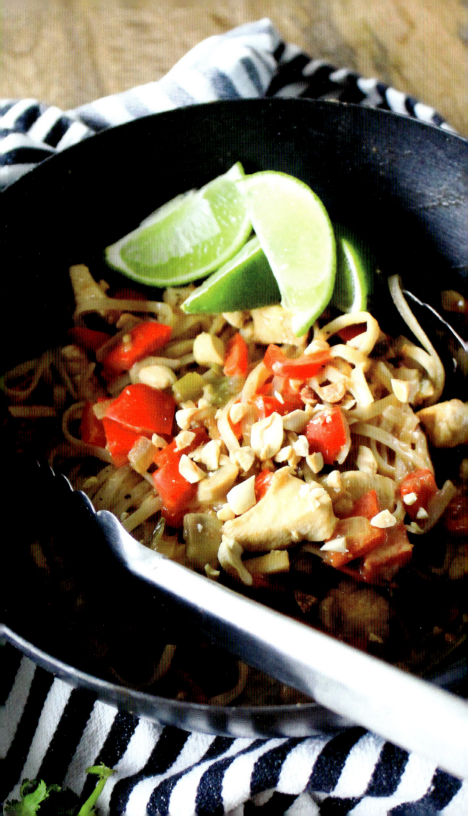

CHICKEN PAD THAI

Makes 4 servings
350 calories / 11F / 36C / 26P / per serving

4 oz. uncooked, pad thai, brown rice noodles
¼ cup OffBeat Sweet Classic Peanut Butter
   or natural peanut butter
¼ cup rice vinegar
2 Tbs. coconut aminos or soy sauce
2 Tbs. raw honey
1 Tbs. fresh, minced garlic
½ cup fresh, minced yellow onion
11 oz. raw chicken breast (8.25 oz. cooked)
2 cups chopped red bell peppers
1 cup sliced green onions
2 cups bean sprouts
Toppings per serving:
5g peanuts
½ lime, juice of
Fresh cilantro
Sea salt and pepper, to taste

1. Cook the noodles according to directions on the package. Drain and set aside.

2. Whisk peanut butter, rice vinegar, coconut aminos and honey in a bowl. If sauce is too thick, add a little water; set aside.

3. Spray a skillet with cooking spray and add the minced garlic and onions. Chop the chicken and add to the skillet. Cook until all the sides are golden brown and the chicken is cooked through.

4. Add the veggies and sauce; cook until tender. Add the noodles last. Weigh the entire recipe and divide by four to get the amount needed to fill one serving. Garnish each serving with the toppings listed. Season with salt and pepper to taste.

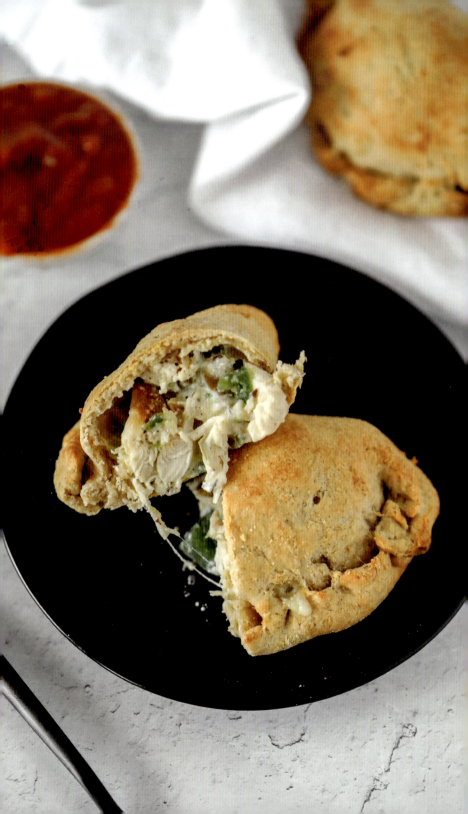

ITALIAN CALZONES

Makes 4 servings
340 calories / 13F / 31C / 24P / per serving

---

5 oz. cooked chicken breast (6.6 oz. raw)
¼ cup chopped mushrooms
¼ cup chopped green bell pepper
2 Tbs. fresh, minced yellow onion
1 ½ cups Kodiak Cakes Buttermillk Mix
2 Tbs. olive oil
6 Tbs. hot water
6 Tbs. part skim, ricotta cheese
6 Tbs. low-fat, shredded mozzarella cheese
Dash of Italian seasoning
1 beaten egg white
½ cup marinara sauce

1. Preheat oven to 400 degrees.

2. Cook the chicken according to the directions in the Food Prep Guide; shred and set aside.

3. Place the mushrooms, bell peppers and onions in a greased pan and sauté until tender, about three minutes. Remove from heat and let cool.

4. Combine the Kodiak Cakes Mix, olive oil and water together. Knead with hands until well combined and smooth. If too dry, add a little bit more water. Place on a baking sheet lined with parchment paper. Cut dough in half, then roll out into two thin circles.

5. Combine the cooked chicken, ricotta cheese, mozzarella cheese and Italian seasoning. Add the veggies and stir until well combined. Split the mixture evenly between both pieces of dough. Fold one side of the dough over the mixture then roll and pinch the edges tight until sealed. Brush tops of the calzones with egg white.

6. Bake for 10-12 minutes or until golden brown. Slice each calzone in half for one serving. Use two tablespoons of marinara sauce for dipping per serving.

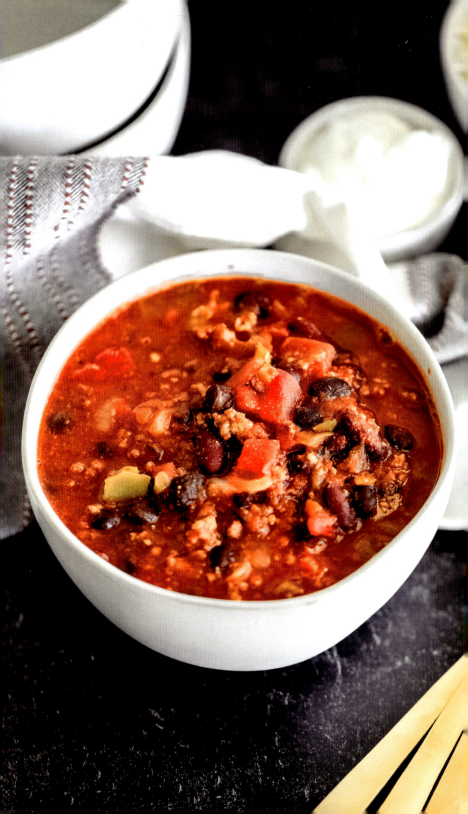

BEST EVER CHILI
Makes 4 servings
350 calories / 12F / 36C / 24P / per serving

8 oz. raw, lean ground beef
1 cup fresh, minced yellow onion
2 cups minced green bell pepper
1 tsp. fresh, minced garlic
2 Tbs. chopped flat leaf parsley
1 chopped jalapeño pepper, optional
2 tsp. ground chili powder
1 tsp. ground cumin
½ tsp. dried oregano
½ tsp. sea salt
½ tsp. ground black pepper
1 cup tomato sauce
2 cups diced tomatoes
1 cup black beans, drained and rinsed
1 cup kidney beans, drained and rinsed
Toppings per serving:
1 Tbs. low-fat, shredded mozzarella cheese
1 Tbs. nonfat, plain Greek yogurt
30g avocado, chopped

1. In a skillet, brown ground beef until no longer pink. Transfer to a crockpot.

2. Spray the skillet with cooking spray and add the onions, bell peppers, garlic, parsley and jalapeño peppers. Cook over medium heat for about five minutes or until veggies are tender and fragrant. Remove from heat and add all the seasonings.

3. Add all ingredients, except for the toppings, to the crockpot. Cook on low for 3-4 hours (or simmer in a pot on the stovetop for 1 hour).

4. Weigh the entire recipe and divide the weight by four to get the amount needed for one serving. Serve warm topped with cheese, Greek yogurt and avocado.

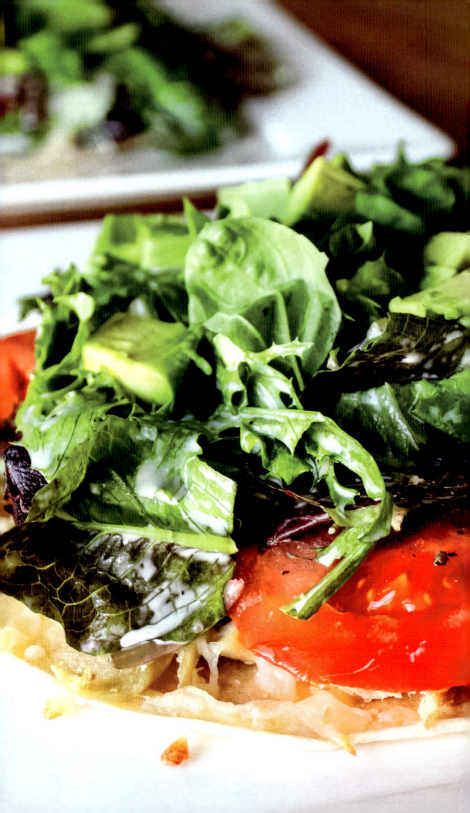

CALIFORNIA CLUB TORTILLA PIZZA

Makes 4 servings
345 calories / 12F / 33C / 26P / per serving

4 oz. cooked chicken breast (5.2 oz. raw)
4 slices turkey bacon, chopped
4 brown rice tortillas
1 cup low-fat, shredded mozzarella cheese
¼ cup low-fat mayo
¼ cup fresh lemon juice
Dash ground black pepper
4 cups baby spring mix salad
2 vine tomatoes, sliced thin
60g avocado, sliced thin
Fresh basil, chopped

1. Preheat oven to 350 degrees.

2. Cook the chicken according to the directions in the Food Prep Guide. Shred and set aside.

3. Add the chopped bacon to a pan or skillet over medium-high heat. Cook until crispy.

4. Place the tortillas on a baking sheet lined with parchment paper. Layer one slice chopped bacon, ¼ of the shredded chicken and ¼ cup cheese to each tortilla. Bake for 10 minutes or until the cheese is melted and lightly brown.

5. While baking, combine the mayo, lemon juice and pepper in a small bowl. Toss with spring salad mix.

6. Top each tortilla pizza with sliced tomatoes, 15g sliced avocado, ¼ of the salad and fresh basil.

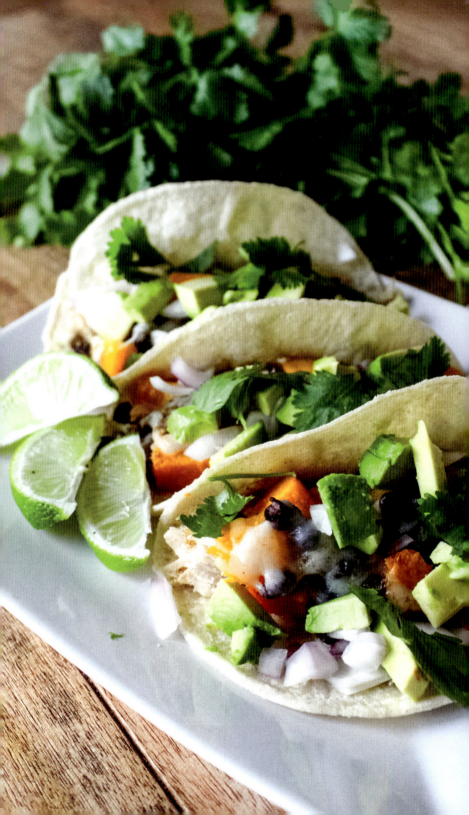

BLACK BEAN & ROASTED BUTTERNUT TACOS
Makes 4 servings
335 calories / 11F / 34C / 25P / per serving

10 oz. raw chicken breasts (7.5 oz. cooked)
½ cup butternut squash, peeled, cubed
8 corn tortillas
8 Tbs. black beans, drained and rinsed
Dash of ground cumin
Dash of sea salt
Dash ground black pepper
8 Tbs. low-fat, shredded mozzarella cheese
8 Tbs. thinly sliced red onion
160g chopped avocado
Cilantro, for garnish
Lime juice, for garnish

1. Cook chicken according to the directions in the Food Prep Guide. Cube and the roast butternut squash according to the directions in the Food Prep Guide.

2. Lay the tortillas out on a baking sheet. Add ⅛ of the chicken, ⅛ of the butternut squash, one tablespoon black beans, seasonings and one tablespoon cheese to the middle of each tortilla. Broil on HI for 3 minutes or until cheese is melted.

3. Top each taco with one tablespoon red onion, 20g avocado, cilantro and lime juice. Enjoy two tacos per serving.

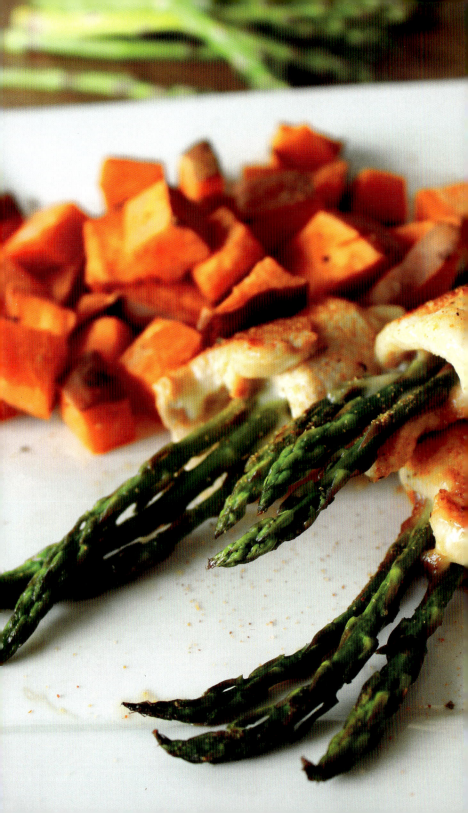

PEPPER JACK CHICKEN WRAPPED ASPARAGUS

Makes 4 servings
350 calories / 12F / 32C / 28P / per serving

460g sweet potatoes, cubed
10 oz. raw chicken breasts (7.5 oz cooked)
6 slices Pepper Jack cheese
36 asparagus spears
Dash of all-purpose seasoning
4 Tbs. Dijon mustard

1. Cube and roast sweet potatoes according to the directions in the Food Prep Guide.

2. Slice the chicken into 12 thin strips (pound flat if needed). Cut cheese slices in half and place one on each chicken strip. Wrap chicken and cheese around three asparagus spears and place seam down in a skillet over medium heat. Sprinkle with seasoning. Cover and cook for five minutes per side or until chicken is cooked through.

3. Enjoy three chicken wraps warm topped with one tablespoon Dijon mustard and ¼ of the roasted sweet potatoes on the side per serving.

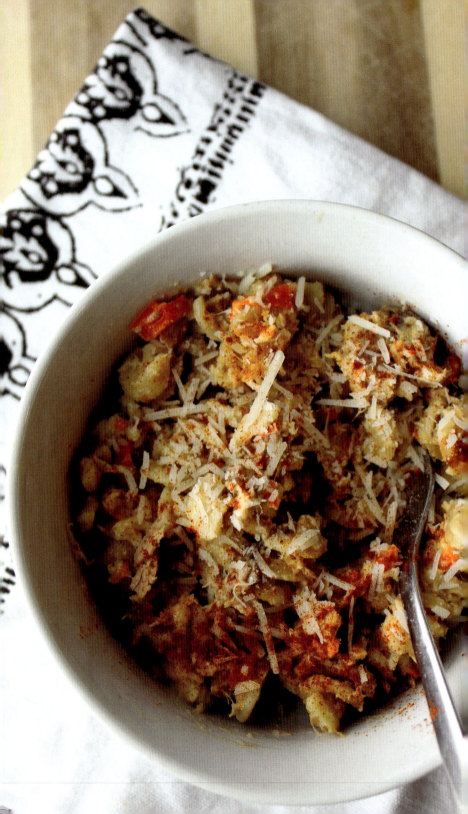

HEARTY TUNA CASSEROLE

Makes 4 servings
350 calories / 11F / 36C / 26P / per serving

5 oz. uncooked whole-wheat fusilli pasta
10 oz. canned tuna, drained
1 cup chopped mushrooms
1 cup chopped red bell peppers
2 Tbs. grass-fed butter
4 Tbs. minced yellow onion
3 Tbs. Kodiak Cakes Buttermilk Mix
½ cup chicken broth
½ cup unsweetened almond milk
Dash of sea salt
Dash of pepper
2 Tbs. olive oil mayo
2 tsp. Dijon mustard
2 Tbs. grated Parmesan cheese
Dash of paprika

1. Preheat oven to 400 degrees.

2. Cook the pasta according to the directions on the package; drain.

3. Combine the pasta, tuna, mushrooms and bell peppers in a bowl; set aside.

4. In a small saucepan, melt butter over medium-low heat. Once melted add the onions and sauté for 1-2 minutes. Whisk in Kodiak Cakes and let cook another 1-2 minutes. Slowly stir in chicken broth and milk. Bring to a boil, stirring continually. Once it begins to boil, turn heat down to low and continue to whisk until the sauce thickens. Remove from heat and season with salt and pepper.

5. Add the mayo and mustard to the sauce. Pour over pasta, tuna and veggies. Stir gently until well combined. Transfer to a greased 8x8 baking dish. Sprinkle parmesan cheese and paprika over the top. Bake for 25 minutes. Slice into four equal portions. Enjoy warm.

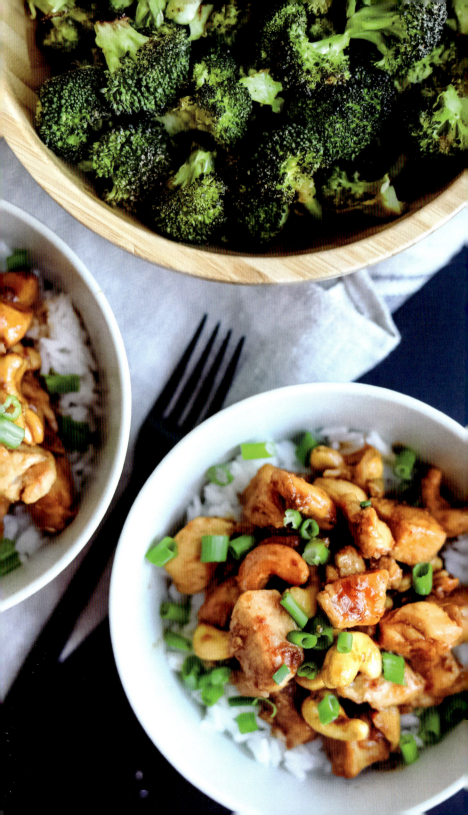

CASHEW KUNG PAO CHICKEN

Makes 4 servings
345 calories / 11F / 35C / 26P / per serving

---

1 cup cooked (⅓ cup uncooked) white or brown jasmine rice
2 cups broccoli florets
12 oz. raw chicken breast (9 oz. cooked)
3 garlic cloves
Dash of ground ginger
3 oz. cashews
Green onions, sliced for garnish

Sweet & Spicy Kung Pao Sauce:
4 Tbs. coconut aminos or soy sauce
2 Tbs. raw honey
1 tsp. Sriracha sauce or chili paste
½ tsp. sesame oil

1. Cook rice according to the directions on the package. Roast broccoli according to directions in the Food Prep Guide.

2. Cube chicken and place in a greased skillet over medium heat. Add whole garlic cloves and ginger. Cook until all sides of the chicken are golden brown and chicken is cooked through. Add the cashews and cook another minute. Turn heat off or down to low heat.

3. Whisk all the sauce ingredients together and add to the skillet. Stir until all the chicken is well coated. Weigh the chicken mixture and divide by four to get the amount needed to fill one serving. Serve one portion of chicken over ¼ cup of cooked rice and garnish with green onions. Enjoy the roasted broccoli on the side or stir in with the chicken and rice.

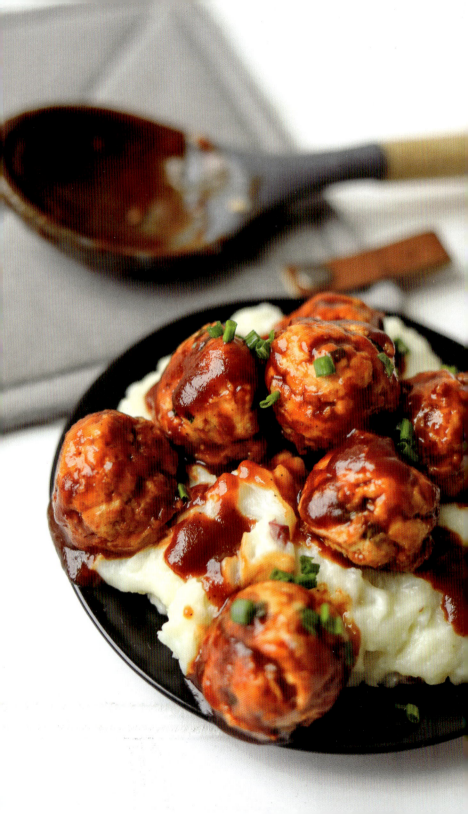

MEATBALLS & MASHED POTATOES

Makes 4 servings
350 calories / 11.5F / 34C / 28P / per serving

1 slice Ezekiel Bread or Harper's Bran Bread
12 oz. raw lean ground turkey
¼ cup yellow onions, minced
4 Tbs. chives
1 tsp. garlic powder
Sea salt and pepper, to taste
½ cup Stubb's BBQ Sauce
12 oz. petite gold potatoes
4 cups cauliflower florets
6 Tbs. nonfat, plain Greek yogurt
½ cup low-fat, mozzarella cheese, shredded
1 Tbs. grass-fed butter

1. Place the bread in a toaster and toast until lightly browned. Break into pieces and place in a blender. Pulse until bread is broken up into crumbs. Mix thawed ground turkey, breadcrumbs, onions, chives, garlic powder, salt and pepper in a bowl.

2. Heat a skillet to medium heat. Scoop the turkey mixture into balls. Spray skillet with cooking spray and add the meatballs. Flip every few minutes until all the sides are browned and the meatballs are fully cooked through. You can also bake the meatballs in the oven at 375 for 15-20 minutes. Add the BBQ sauce to the meatballs and stir until the meatballs are coated. Turn heat off; cover to keep warm.

3. Bring a pot of water to a boil. Add potatoes. Boil for 10 minutes. Add cauliflower to the pot with the potatoes and boil for another 10 minutes. Drain and remove from heat.

4. Add the Greek yogurt, cheese, butter, salt, pepper and a dash of garlic powder to the potatoes and cauliflower. Beat with a hand mixer until smooth and creamy.

5. Weigh the meatballs and the mashed potatoes separately, then divide the weight by four to get the amount needed to fill one serving. Serve meatballs over mashed potatoes.

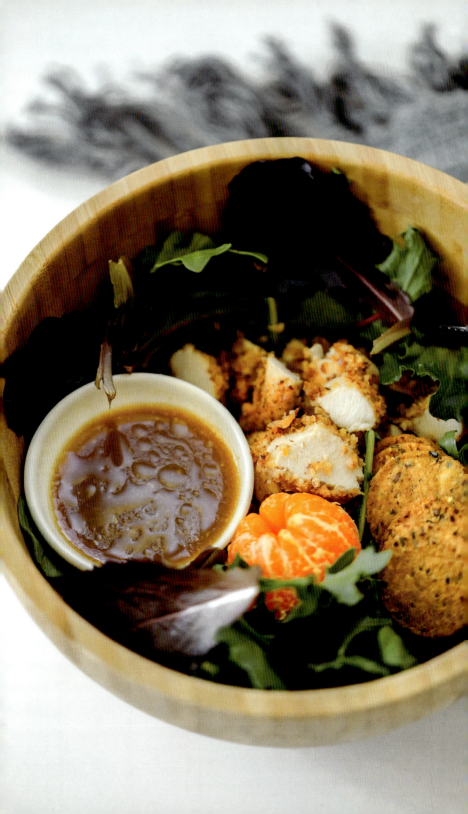

ORANGE ALMOND CHICKEN SALAD

Makes 4 servings
340 calories / 12F / 33C / 25P / per serving

---

12 oz. raw chicken tenderloins (9 oz. cooked)
¼ cup chopped almonds
¼ cup whole-wheat bread crumbs
Dash of all-purpose seasoning
8 cups spring lettuce mix
Orange Balsamic Marinade:
½ cup Simply Orange Juice
2 Tbs. balsamic vinegar
1 Tbs. olive oil
1 Tbs. raw honey
1 Tbs. Dijon mustard
Toppings per serving:
1 clementine orange, peeled and halved
6 sweet potato crackers, crumbled

1. Add all of the ingredients for the marinade to a bowl. Whisk until well combined. Weigh the marinade and divide in half. Marinate chicken in ½ of the marinade for 2+ hours. Reserve the remaining marinade in the fridge to use for the salad dressing.

2. Preheat oven to 375 degrees.

3. Combine the chopped almonds, bread crumbs and seasoning. Dip the chicken into the mixture and place on a baking sheet lined with parchment paper. Discard the used marinade. Bake for 15-20 minutes or until cooked through.

4. Place ¼ of the chicken on top of two cups of the spring lettuce mix. Weigh the remaining Orange Balsamic Marinade and divide the weight by four to get the amount needed to fill one serving. Drizzle each salad with one serving of dressing, then top with orange slices and cracker crumbles.

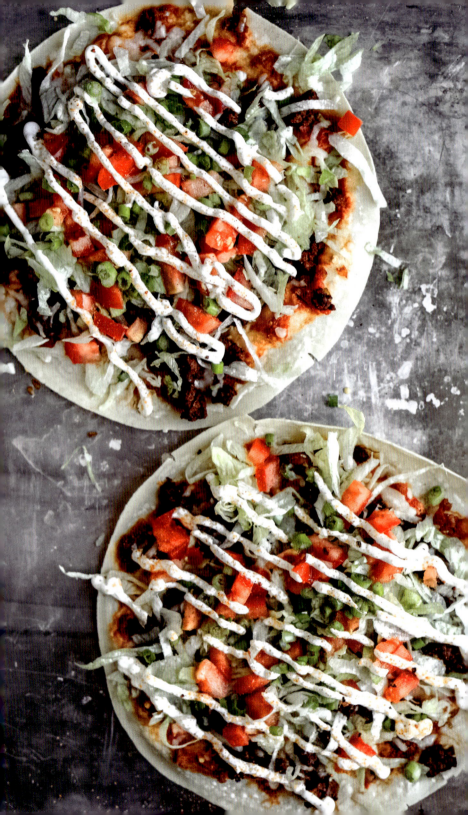

MEXICAN TORTILLA PIZZA
Makes 4 serving
330 calories / 12F / 31C / 24P / per serving

10 oz. raw lean ground beef
3 Tbs. taco seasoning
4 brown rice tortillas
8 Tbs. salsa
12 Tbs. low-fat, shredded mozzarella cheese
4 cups shredded lettuce
1 cup fresh vine tomatoes, diced
4 Tbs. green onions, chopped
4 Tbs. nonfat, plain Greek yogurt

1. Preheat the oven 350 degrees.

2. Brown the ground beef in a pan over medium heat. Once cooked through, add the taco seasoning. Remove from heat.

3. Lay the tortillas out flat on a baking sheet and spread two table-spoons salsa over the top of each one. Add three tablespoons of cheese and ¼ of the cooked ground beef to each tortilla.

4. Bake for 10 minutes or until the cheese is melted. Top each serving with one cup shredded lettuce, ¼ cup fresh tomatoes, one tablespoon plain Greek yogurt and one tablespoon of sliced green onions.

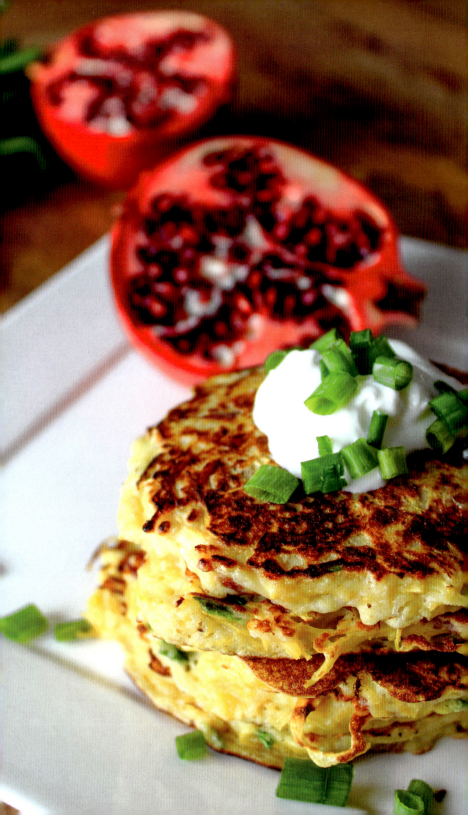

SPAGHETTI SQUASH & BACON FRITTERS

Makes 4 servings
350 calories / 12.5F / 32C / 27.5P / per serving

6 cups roasted spaghetti squash
4 slices turkey bacon
4 large eggs
⅔ cup Kodiak Cakes Buttermilk Mix
¾ cup grated Parmesan cheese
6 chopped green onions
½ tsp. sea salt
Toppings per serving:
1 Tbs. nonfat, plain Greek yogurt
1 Tbs. fresh salsa
1 Tbs. green onions, chopped
Side per serving:
25 grams pomegranate seeds

1. Roast spaghetti squash according to directions in the Food Prep Guide. Once cooled, place squash in a paper towel and wring out the liquid with your hands over the sink. Try to get as much of the liquid out as you can.

2. Chop the bacon and cook it in a frying pan over medium-high heat until crispy; set aside.

3. Beat the eggs with an electric mixture on high for 2 minutes. Add the Kodiak Cakes Mix and beat until well combined. Add the spaghetti squash, Parmesan cheese, green onion, bacon and sea salt. Mix until well combined.

4. Heat a skillet to medium-high heat. Once hot, spray with cooking spray and spoon ¼ cup of the mixture onto the skillet. Shape and flatten the top so the fritter is level. Repeat with the remaining mixture. Cook until the bottom side is golden brown, then flip the fritter over. Once both sides are golden brown, remove from the pan and top with Greek yogurt, salsa and green onions. Enjoy pomegranate seeds on the side.

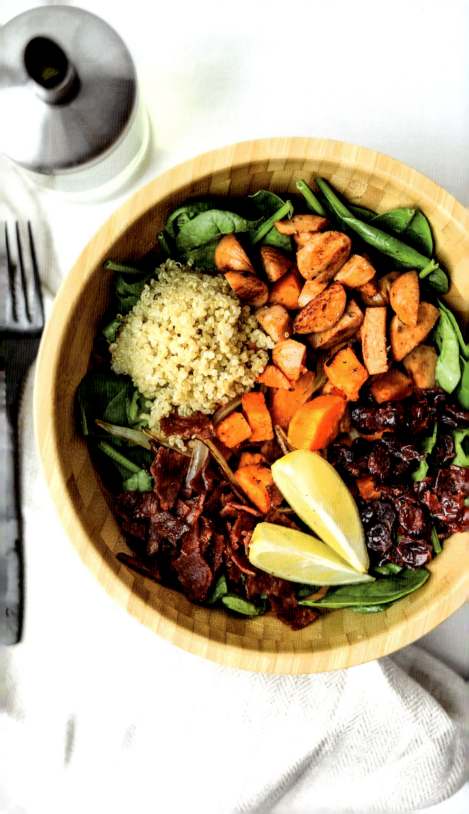

ROASTED BUTTERNUT SQUASH & QUINOA SALAD

Makes 4 servings
340 calories / 12F / 34C / 24P / per serving

2 chicken sausage links, sliced into rounds
8 slices turkey bacon, chopped
20 oz. raw butternut squash, peeled and diced
½ of a sweet onion, thinly sliced
1 cup cooked (⅓ cup uncooked) quinoa
2 Tbs. fresh lemon juice
1 Tbs. olive oil
Stevia in the Raw, to taste
Sea salt, to taste
4 cups chopped spinach
4 Tbs. dried unsweetened cranberries

1. Preheat oven to 425 degrees and line a baking sheet with parchment paper.

2. Chop the sausage, turkey bacon and butternut squash. Thinly slice the sweet onion. Pour them onto the baking sheet. Spray tops with cooking spray and sprinkle with sea salt. Roast in the oven for 20-25 minutes or until the squash is tender.

3. Cook the quinoa according to directions on package.

4. Whisk the lemon juice, olive oil, stevia and a pinch of salt together in a small bowl to make the dressing; set aside.

5. Combine the butternut squash, onions, sausage and quinoa together in a bowl. Stir in the spinach and cranberries. Add the dressing and toss until well coated. Weigh entire recipe and divide the weight by four to get the amount needed to fill one serving. Enjoy warm.

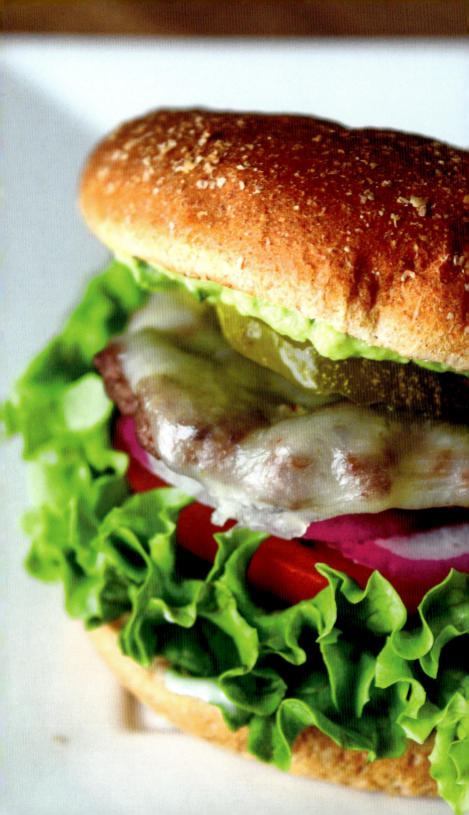

PEPPER JACK BISON BURGERS

Makes 4 serving
360 calories / 14F / 31C / 27P / per serving

12 oz. lean ground bison
Sea salt and pepper, to taste
2 oz. Pepper Jack cheese, shredded
4 whole wheat hamburger buns (140 cals each)
4 Tbs. ketchup
Mustard, optional
4 Dill pickles
4 slices red onion
4 tomato slices
4 butter lettuce leaves

1. Preheat oven to HI broil.

2. Combine the ground bison with salt and pepper. Form into four, three ounce patties. Line a rimmed baking sheet with foil, then spray with cooking spray. Place the patties on the baking sheet. Broil in the oven on the middle rack for 5-6 minutes per side. Add ½ ounce of cheese to each patty and broil another 1-2 minutes until the cheese is melted.

3. Toast buns if desired. Spread one tablespoon of ketchup on each bun; add mustard if desired. Add burger patties and remaining toppings to the middle. Enjoy!

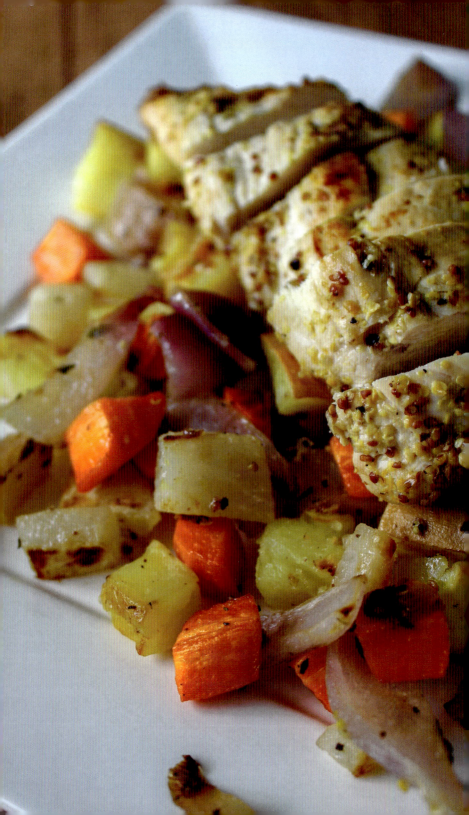

MUSTARD ROASTED CHICKEN & VEGGIES

Makes 4 servings
350 calories / 12F / 34C / 26P / per serving

14 oz. raw chicken breast (10.5 oz. cooked)
2 Tbs. whole-grain mustard
1 Tbs. coconut aminos or soy sauce
Dash of ground black pepper
16 oz. sweet potatoes, cubed
8 oz. peeled and diced turnips
8 oz. peeled and diced carrots
1 cup red onion, cut into wedges
3 Tbs. olive oil
2 sprigs of fresh thyme
Sea salt and pepper, to taste

1. Preheat oven to 400 degrees.

2. Pat the chicken dry with paper towels. Combine the mustard, coconut aminos and pepper in a bowl. Add the chicken and stir to coat; set aside.

3. Place the sweet potatoes, turnips, carrots, onion, olive oil, thyme, salt and pepper in a large Ziploc bag. Massage until well coated. Pour out onto a roasting pan lined with foil.

4. Add the chicken to veggie pan. Roast until the chicken is cooked through and veggies are tender, about 30-40 minutes. Split veggies into four equal portions and serve with two ounces of chicken. Enjoy warm.

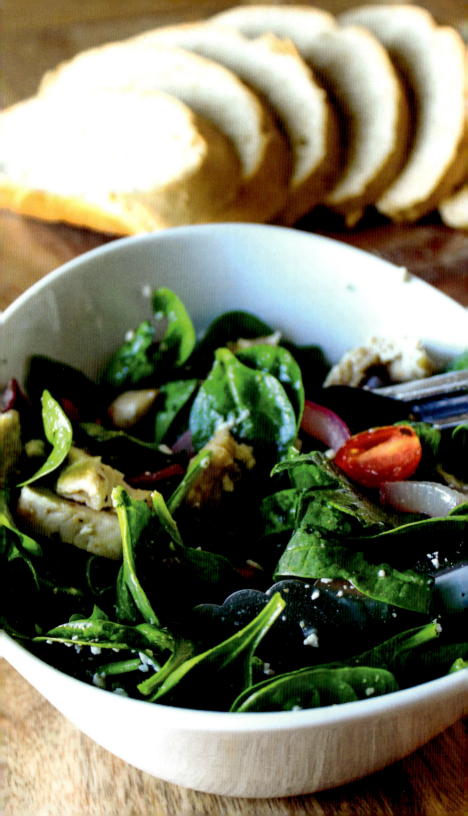

LEMON PEPPER CHICKEN SALAD

Makes 4 servings
335 calories / 11F / 32C / 27P / per serving

4 slices Homemade Honey-Wheat Bread
2 Tbs. olive oil
4 Tbs. fresh lemon juice
Dash of Sriracha sauce
¼ tsp. dried thyme
Sea salt
Ground black pepper
10 oz. raw chicken breast (7.5 oz. cooked)
1 cup red onion, sliced into rings
¼ tsp. lemon pepper
8 cups chopped spinach
1 cup cherry tomatoes, halved
4 Tbs. feta cheese crumbles

1. Make the Homemade Honey-Wheat Bread in advance. Recipe in the Food Prep Guide.

2. Whisk the olive oil, lemon juice, Sriracha and thyme in a small saucepan over low heat. Add salt and pepper to taste. Remove from heat and keep warm. Weigh the dressing and divide the weight by four to get the amount needed to fill one serving.

3. Heat oven to HI broil. Place the chicken and onions onto a greased broiler pan. Sprinkle with sea salt and lemon pepper. Broil for 8 minutes per side. Cut the chicken crosswise into thin slices. Separate the onions into rings.

4. For each serving, layer 2 cups of spinach, ¼ warm chicken, ¼ cup onions, ¼ cup tomatoes and ¼ of the warm dressing. Toss and top with 1 tablespoon feta cheese. Enjoy one serving of the home-made bread on the side.

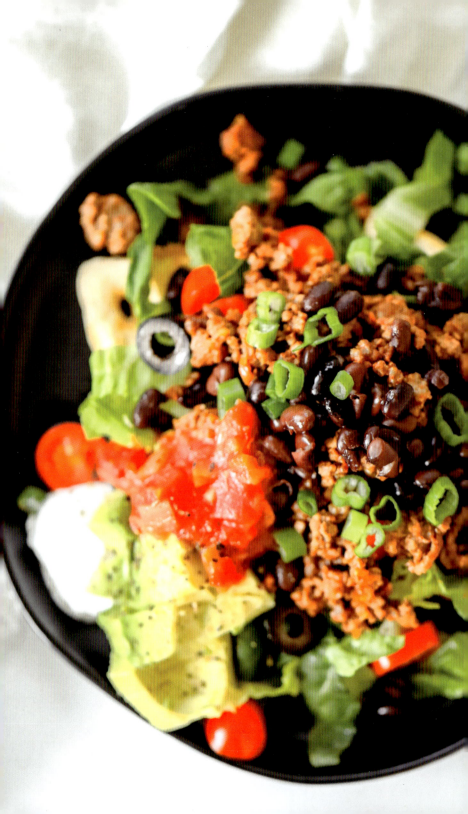

WAFFLED NAVAJO TACO

Makes 4 servings
350 calories / 12F / 34C / 26P / per serving

8 oz. lean ground beef
2 Tbs. taco seasoning
1 ½ cups Kodiak Cakes Buttermilk Mix
1 cup water
½ cup black beans, drained and rinsed
4 cups shredded green leaf lettuce
1 cup cherry tomatoes, halved

Toppings per serving:
1 Tbs. nonfat, plain Greek yogurt
1 Tbs. salsa
1 Tbs. green onions
½ Tbs. sliced olives
25g chopped avocado

1. Brown the ground beef in a frying pan over medium-high heat. Once browned, add taco seasoning. Remove from heat and keep warm.

2. Heat waffle iron. Combine Kodiak Cakes Mix and water. Spray waffle iron and pour ¼ of the batter onto the waffle iron. Repeat.

3. Top each waffle with ¼ of the browned ground beef, two tablespoons black beans, 1 cup lettuce, ¼ cup tomatoes and all other toppings listed per serving.

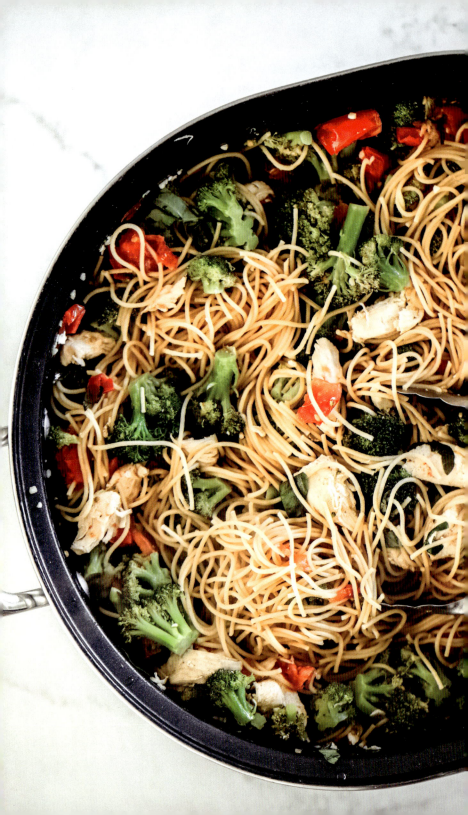

TOMATO BUTTER CHICKEN SPAGHETTI

Makes 4 servings
350 calories / 11F / 34C / 28P / per serving

4.5 oz. uncooked whole wheat spaghetti
12 oz. raw chicken breast (9 oz. cooked)
Sea salt
Ground black pepper
4 vine tomatoes, diced
1 tsp. minced garlic
A pinch of fresh basil
1 Tbs. olive oil
4 cups raw broccoli, chopped
2 Tbs. grass-fed butter

1. Cook spaghetti according to directions on package; drain.
Weigh the spaghetti and divide the weight by four to get the
amount needed to fill one serving.

2. Butterfly-cut the chicken to make it even in thickness. Sprinkle
both sides with sea salt and pepper. Dice tomatoes, mince the
garlic and chop the basil.

3. Heat the oil in a skillet over medium heat. Add the chicken.
Cover and cook for about 3 - 4 minutes per side or until cooked
through. Turn heat down and remove chicken; set aside.

4. Let the oil cool. Add the tomatoes and broccoli to the skillet and
turn the heat back up to medium. Break up the tomatoes and simmer for about 4 minutes. Add the garlic and butter; stir to combine
until the butter is melted. Add the chicken back to the pan and
let marinate for a few minutes. Weigh the tomato butter chicken
mixture, then divide the weight by four to get the amount needed
to fill one serving.

5. Top one serving of spaghetti with one serving of the tomato
butter chicken mixture. Top with fresh basil and season with sea salt
and pepper, to taste.

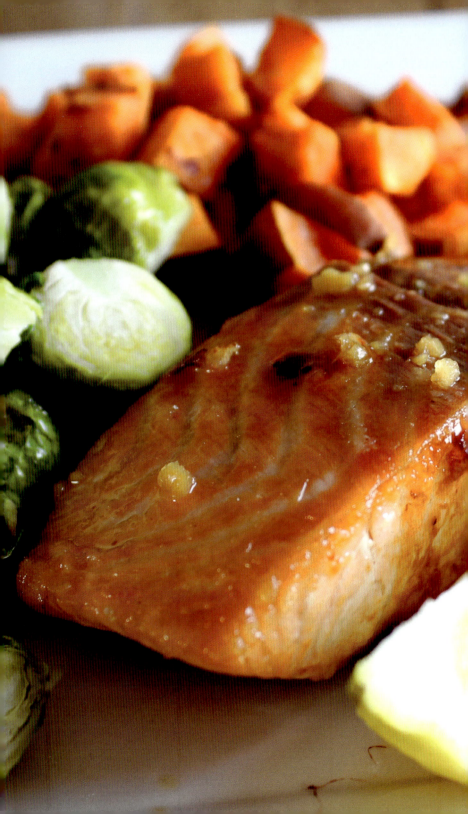

HONEY GARLIC SALMON
Makes 4 servings
335 calories / 11F / 35C / 24P / per serving

16 oz. sweet potatoes
4 cups Brussels sprouts
12 oz. wild caught salmon
Sea salt and pepper, to taste
2 Tbs. olive oil
½ tsp. fresh, minced garlic
2 Tbs. raw honey
1 Tbs. fresh lemon juice
Parsley for garnish, optional

1. Cube the sweet potatoes. Trim and halve the Brussels sprouts. Roast both according to directions in the Food Prep Guide.

2. While the veggies are roasting, prepare the salmon. Sprinkle the salmon with sea salt and pepper. Add the oil to a large skillet over medium heat. Once hot, add the salmon to the skillet skin side down. Cover and cook for five minutes. Whisk the honey, lemon juice and garlic together in a small bowl. Carefully flip the salmon over and cook for five more minutes or until salmon is fully cooked and begins to flake. Remove the skin. Add the honey, lemon, garlic mixture to the pan for the last minute.

3. Serve ¼ of salmon alongside ¼ of roasted sweet potatoes and ¼ of the Brussels sprouts. Garnish with chopped parsley.

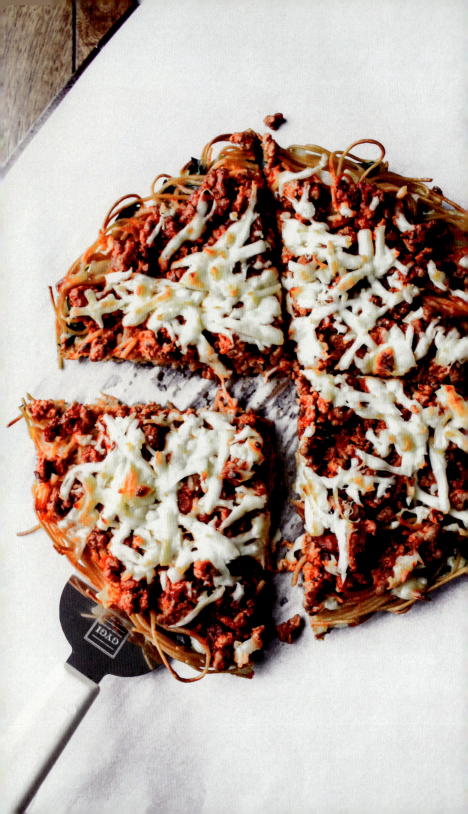

SPAGHETTI PIZZA PIE

Makes 4 servings
345 calories / 11F / 33C / 28P / per serving

5 oz. uncooked whole grain spaghetti
½ cup chopped yellow onions
½ tsp. fresh, minced garlic
1 cup chopped spinach
½ cup low-fat cottage cheese
2 large eggs, beaten
8 oz. lean ground turkey
1 cup marinara sauce
½ cup low-fat, shredded mozzarella cheese

1. Preheat oven to 350 degrees. Cook the spaghetti according to the directions on the package.

2. Spray a frying pan with cooking spray and sauté the onions, garlic and spinach over medium heat until the onions are tender. Add the cottage cheese and cook until melted. Remove from heat and place in a bowl.

3. Add the cooked spaghetti and beaten egg to the bowl, stir until well combined. Press into two greased 9" pie pans to form a crust.

4. Brown the turkey in a pan over med/high heat. Combine cooked ground turkey and marinara sauce, then spread evenly over the spaghetti crusts. Sprinkle cheese on top and bake for 30 minutes. Let stand for five minutes, then cut each pie into four slices and serve warm.

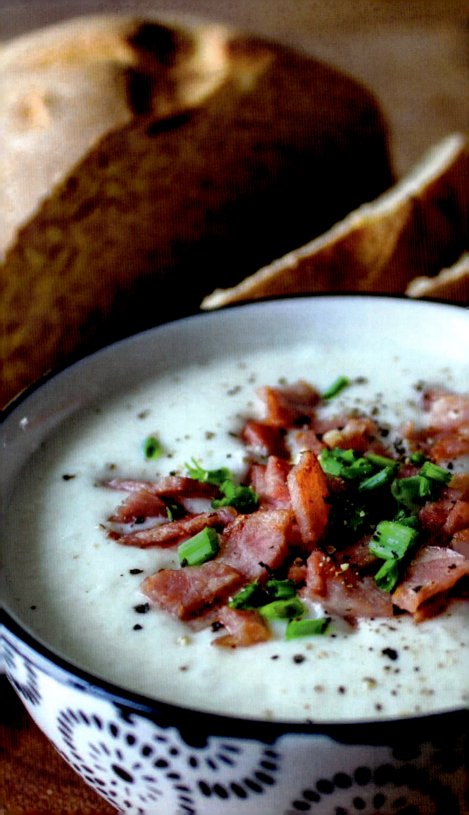

ROASTED CAULIFLOWER SOUP

Makes 4 servings
325 calories / 10.5F / 31.5C / 26P / per serving

4 slices (8 oz.) Homemade Honey-Wheat Bread
4 cups cauliflower florets
½ cup chopped yellow onion
½ tsp. fresh, minced garlic
1 Tbs. olive oil
2 cups chicken bone broth
⅔ cup low-fat, shredded mozzarella cheese
⅔ cup nonfat, plain Greek yogurt
Sea salt and pepper, to taste
4 slices chopped turkey bacon
Chives, for garnish

1. Make the Homemade Honey-Wheat Bread in advance. Recipe in the Food Prep Guide.

2. Preheat oven to 400 degrees.

3. Add the cauliflower florets, onion, garlic and olive oil to a large Ziploc bag. Massage until well coated. Spread out onto a baking sheet lined with parchment paper and roast for 20 minutes.

4. Spray a frying pan and place over medium heat. Add chopped bacon to the pan and cook until crispy. Remove from pan and set aside.

5. Add roasted cauliflower and onions, chicken broth, mozzarella cheese, Greek yogurt, salt and pepper to a blender. Blend on high until smooth. Weigh the soup and divide the weight by four to get the amount needed for one serving.

6. Top each serving of soup with one slice crumbled bacon and chives. Enjoy with 2 oz. homemade bread on the side.

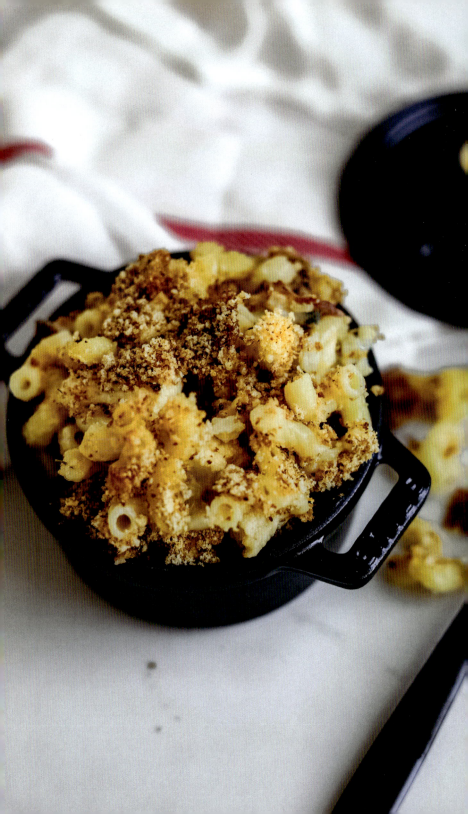

BOSS BAKED MAC & CHEESE

Makes 4 servings
350 calories / 14.5F / 31.5C / 23.5P / per serving

---

3 cups cauliflower florets
4 oz. uncooked whole wheat macaroni or elbow pasta
1 Italian chicken sausage
2 slices turkey bacon
1 Tbs. grass-fed butter
1 Tbs. Kodiak Cakes Buttermilk Mix
1 cup fat-free milk
¼ tsp. sea salt
Dash of ground black pepper
½ cup low-fat, shredded cheddar cheese
6 Tbs. grated Parmesan cheese
1 slice Ezekiel bread
Dash of sea salt, garlic powder, paprika, thyme

1. Heat oven to 350 degrees.

2. Bake cauliflower according to the directions in the Food Prep Guide. Cook macaroni according to the directions on the package. Drain and set aside.

3. Slice the chicken sausage into thin rounds and chop bacon into small pieces. Place in a frying pan over medium/high heat. Cook until fragrant and all sides are browned. Remove from heat and set aside.

4. In a large saucepan, melt the butter over low/medium heat. Add the Kodiak Cakes Mix and stir until well combined. Slowly whisk in the milk and stir constantly until slightly thickened. Add in the sea salt, black pepper, cheddar cheese and four tablespoons of the Parmesan cheese. Stir until the cheese is melted into the sauce. Add the cauliflower, macaroni, sausage and bacon to the sauce. Stir until well combined. Pour into an 8x8 baking dish.

5. Toast the Ezekiel bread in the toaster until browned on both sides. Break into pieces and place in a blender. Pulse until it turns into bread crumbs. Combine the bread crumbs, two tablespoons Parmesan cheese, sea salt, garlic powder, paprika and thyme together in a bowl. Sprinkle over the top of the macaroni. Bake for 25 minutes. Divide into four equal servings and enjoy warm.

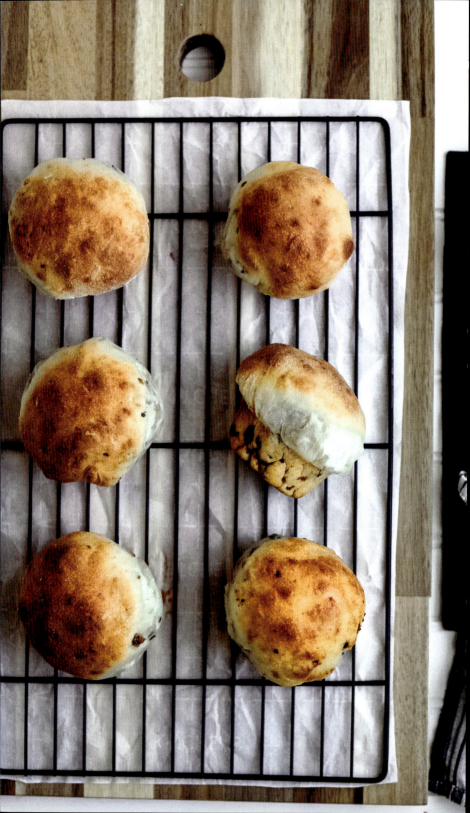

SUPREME PIZZA POPOVERS

Makes 4 servings
345 calories / 10.5F / 37C / 25P / per serving

---

6 oz. raw lean ground turkey
½ tsp. fresh minced garlic
½ tsp. Italian seasoning
¼ tsp. dried parsley
¼ tsp. sea salt
¼ tsp. dried minced onion
⅛ tsp. ground black pepper
⅛ tsp. paprika
Pinch of fennel seeds
Pinch of red pepper flakes

½ cup chopped mushrooms
½ cup chopped green bell peppers
¼ cup chopped red onions
¼ cup sliced black olives
1 ¼ cup self-rising flour
⅔ cup nonfat, plain Greek yogurt
1 Tbs. water
1 cup low-fat, shredded mozzarella
   cheese
½ cup traditional pizza sauce

1. Preheat oven to 450 degrees.

2. Add the ground turkey to a greased skillet. Cook over medium heat until browned. Add all the seasonings and stir until well combined. Chop the veggies, then add them to the skillet with the turkey; cook until tender. Transfer to a bowl and weigh the mixture. Divide the weight by four to get the amount needed for one serving.

3. Place the self-rising flour, Greek yogurt and water into a mixing bowl. Knead until well combined. If the dough is too dry, add a little water. Weigh the dough and divide it into four equal balls. Flatten each ball and roll out thin into a circle.

4. Place ¼ cup of the cheese into the middle of each dough round and fill with one serving of the turkey mixture. Fold the edges of the dough up over the top of the mixture and pinch together. Place the popovers seam down into the muffin tin. Bake for 15-20 minutes. Enjoy one popover per serving with two tablespoons pizza sauce.

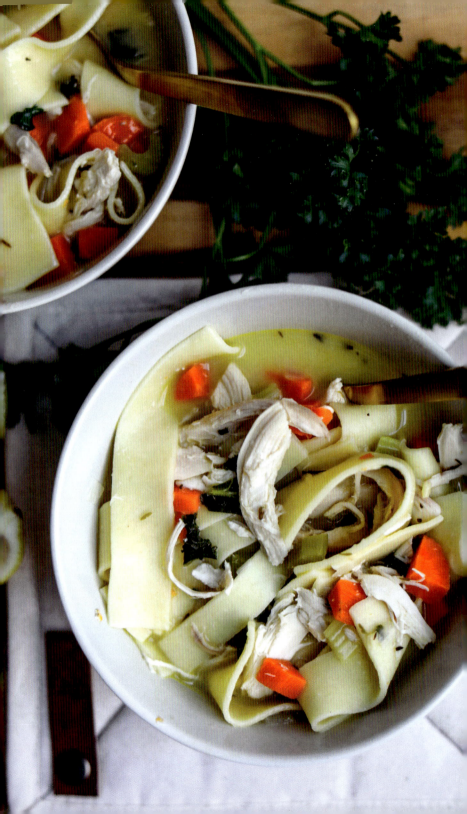

CREAMY CHICKEN NOODLE SOUP

Makes 4 servings
350 calories / 12F / 33C / 27P / per serving

1 Tbs. olive oil
½ cup diced yellow onion
3 cups chicken broth
2 cups water
1 bay leaf
1 tsp. fresh minced garlic
½ tsp. dried thyme
½ tsp. sea salt
1 ½ cups chopped carrots
1 cup chopped celery
1 cup chopped kale
4 oz. uncooked egg noodles
1 Tbs. grass-fed butter
2 Tbs. Kodiak Cakes Buttermilk Mix
¼ cup canned, lite coconut milk
11 oz. rotisserie chicken breast, shredded
½ of a lemon, juice of
2 Tbs. fresh chopped parsley

1. Add the olive oil and diced onion to a large pot over medium heat. Sauté for about 3 minutes or until fragrant and tender. Stir in the chicken broth and water. Add the bay leaf, minced garlic, thyme and sea salt. Bring to a boil and then reduce heat and let simmer for 20 minutes.

2. Add in the carrots, celery and kale. Let cook about five minutes and then add the uncooked egg noodles. Cook the noodles al dente according to the directions on the package.

3. Add the butter to a large frying pan over low heat. Once melted, stir in the Kodiak Cakes Mix. Add one cup of broth from the soup to the pan, then slowly whisk it in along with the coconut milk. Bring to a boil; stirring constantly. Remove from heat and add to the pot of soup once the noodles are done cooking.

4. Add the shredded chicken last and simmer until the chicken is warm. Squeeze lemon juice over the soup and it is ready to serve. Weigh the entire soup and divide the weight by four to get the amount needed for one serving. Garnish each bowl with fresh parsley.

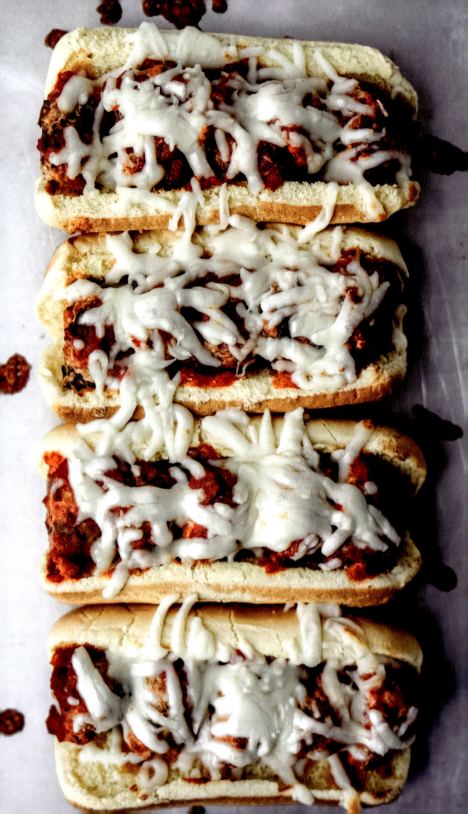

MEATBALL SUBS

Makes 4 servings
350 calories / 11.5F / 33C / 28.5P / per serving

1 slice Ezekiel bread
10 oz. raw lean ground turkey
1 large egg
1 cup finely chopped spinach
½ cup finely chopped red bell peppers
1 Tbs. dried minced onion
1 Tbs. tomato paste
1 tsp. fresh, minced garlic
1 tsp. all-purpose seasoning
¼ tsp. sea salt
Dash of ground black pepper
1 cup marinara sauce
½ cup low-fat, shredded mozzarella cheese
4 whole-wheat or potato hot dog buns

1. Preheat oven to 400 degrees.

2. Toast the bread in a toaster until browned and crispy. Break up into pieces and place in a blender. Pulse into crumbs; set aside.

3. Add the ground turkey, egg, homemade bread crumbs, spinach, bell peppers, onion, tomato paste, garlic and seasonings to a bowl. Mix with hands until well combined. Using a cookie scoop, scoop into 20, 1-inch balls and place in a 9x13 non-stick baking dish. Cover with marinara sauce and bake for 15-20 minutes or until cooked through.

4. Place the hotdog buns on a baking sheet lined with parchment paper. Open the buns and spray the inside lightly with cooking spray. Place in the oven at 350 degrees for 5 minutes to toast the inside.

5. Distribute the meatballs evenly between the four hot dog buns. Top each sub sandwich with two tablespoons mozzarella cheese and return to the oven for 3-5 minutes or until the cheese is melted and the subs are heated through. *Only make the subs that you are going to eat today. The buns will get soggy if the meatballs are left on them too long.

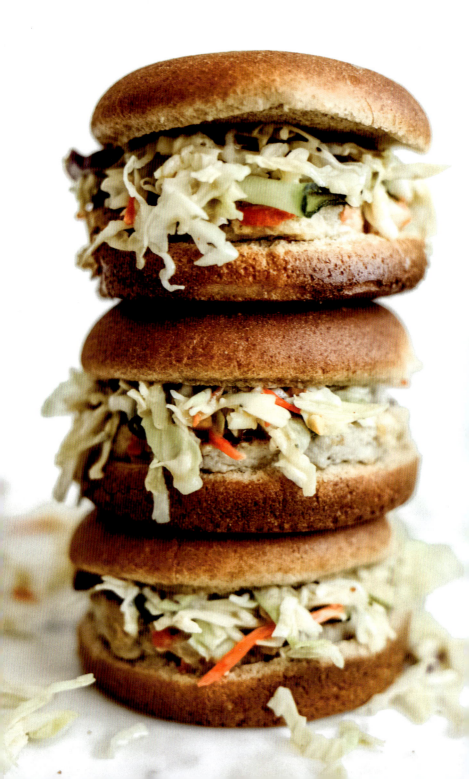

THAI CRUNCH BURGER
Makes 4 servings
350 calories / 12.5F / 35C / 24.5P / per serving

---

12 oz. lean ground turkey
¼ cup finely chopped red bell peppers
¼ cup finely chopped carrots
¼ cup finely chopped yellow onions
1 tsp. fresh grated ginger
½ tsp. sea salt
Thai Peanut Dressing (recipe below)
2 Tbs. Bolthouse Farms Classic Ranch or Cilantro Avocado Dressing
4 cups coleslaw salad mix (without dressing)
12 cucumber slices
4 whole wheat hamburger buns
Thai Peanut Dressing:
1 Tbs. OffBeat Sweet Classic Peanut Butter
   or natural peanut butter
1 Tbs. raw honey
½ Tbs. olive oil
1 tsp. water
1 tsp. rice vinegar
1 tsp. coconut aminos or soy sauce
Dash of sea salt
Dash of cayenne pepper

1. Place the ground turkey in a bowl with the bell peppers, carrots, onions, ginger and sea salt. Mix with hands until well combined. Weigh the mixture and divide into four equal portions. Form into patties and set aside.

2. Heat a grill top or skillet to medium heat. Add the burger patties and cook for about 5-7 minutes per side or until browned and fully cooked through. Transfer to a plate and cover with foil to keep warm.

3. Whisk all of the Thai Peanut Dressing ingredients together in a bowl. Stir in the Bolthouse Farms Dressing. Add the coleslaw mix and stir until well coated.

4. Toast the buns if desired. Place the burgers on the buns and top each one evenly with the slaw and three cucumber slices. Sprinkle salt and pepper over the cucumbers and top with the other half of the bun.

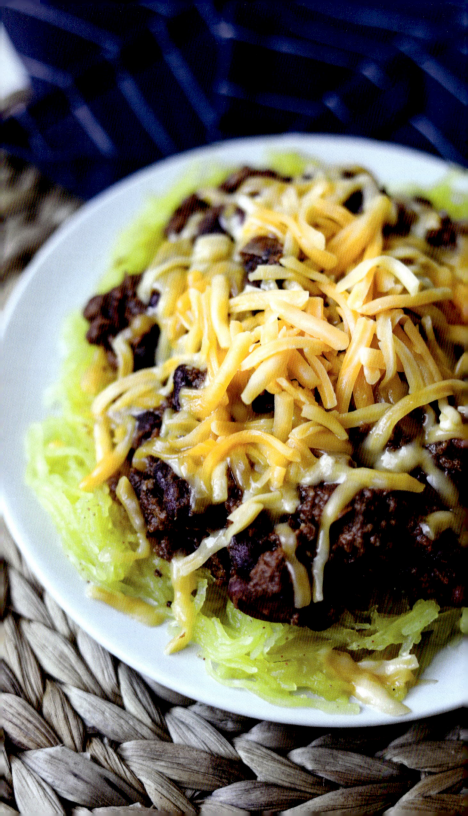

CINCINNATI STYLE CHILI

Make 4 servings
345 calories / 12F / 33C / 26P / per serving

10 oz. lean ground beef
2 cups kidney beans, drained and rinsed
¼ cup diced yellow onions
½ cup tomato sauce
2 Tbs. water
½ Tbs. white wine vinegar
½ tsp. Worcestershire sauce
1 tsp. fresh minced garlic
¼ ounce of unsweetened baking chocolate
1 Tbs. chili powder
¼ tsp. sea salt
¼ tsp. ground cumin
¼ tsp. ground cinnamon
Dash of cayenne pepper
Dash of ground cloves
1 bay leaf
4 cups cooked spaghetti squash
½ cup low-fat, shredded cheddar cheese

1. Place all the ingredients into a crockpot, except for the spaghetti squash and cheese. Cook on low for 6-8 hours or on high for 3-4 hours. Weigh the chili and divide by four to get the amount needed to fill one serving.

2. Cook the spaghetti squash according to the directions in the Food Prep Guide. Rake the cooked spaghetti squash into a bowl and sprinkle with salt and pepper; set aside.

3. Serve by placing one serving of chili over one cup of spaghetti squash. Top each portion with two tablespoons of cheddar cheese.

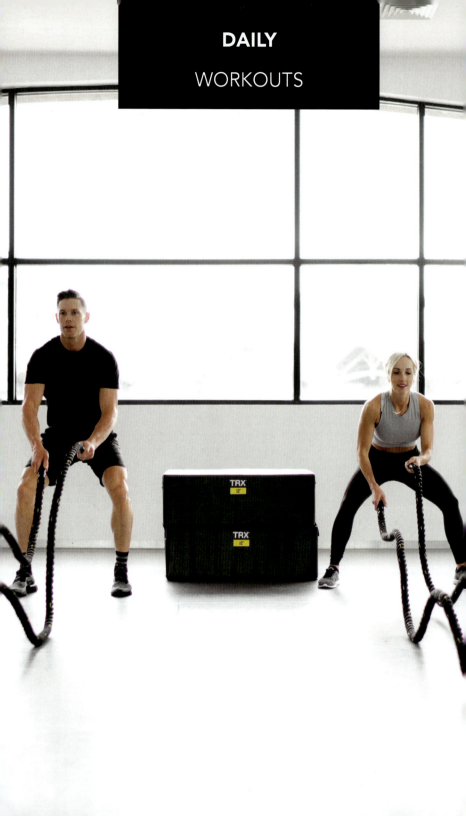

DAILY

WORKOUTS

GOOD THINGS COME TO THOSE WHO SWEAT

HIIT

Set your timer for 30 seconds of work, 15 seconds of rest, 8 cycles. Perform each of the following sets 2 times through. For example… Round 1: Complete 30 seconds of mountain climbers followed by 15 seconds of rest. Now, move to 30 seconds of push-ups followed by 15 seconds of rest. Complete the last two movements and start immediately back at mountain climbers for 1 more cycle! Rest 90 seconds between rounds. **Total time:** 27:30

Warm-up
5 minutes of brisk walking, jogging in place, jumping rope, etc.

ROUND 1	ROUND 2	ROUND 3
MOUNTAIN CLIMBERS	PIKED PUSH-UPS	COMMANDOS
PUSH-UPS	WALKING LUNGES	JUMP SQUATS
JUMPING JACKS	TUCK JUMPS	V-SIT
PLANK	V-UPS	BURPEES

ADVANCED WOD
"THE DIRTY 30"
30 WALL BALLS 20/14
30 TOES TO BAR
30 BURPEES
30 CALORIE ROW
30 THRUSTERS 115/75
30 CALORIE ROW
30 BURPEES
30 TOES TO BAR
30 WALL BALLS

TABATA

Set your timer for 20 seconds of work, 10 seconds of rest, 16 cycles. Perform each of the following paired movements 8 times through. For example… Movement 1: Complete 20 seconds of wall sits followed by 10 seconds of rest. Now, move to exercise #2 for 20 seconds. Rest 10 seconds and you're right back at movement #1. Repeat this pattern through 8 rounds of each movement. Push as hard as you can for 20 seconds through each interval. Rest 90 seconds between rounds. **Total time:** 33:30

Warm-up

5 minutes of brisk walking, jogging in place, jumping rope, etc.

1. WALL SITS   **3.** PLANK   **5.** RUSSIAN TWISTS
2. BURPEES   **4.** JUMP ROPE   **6.** JUMPING LUNGES

ADVANCED WOD
"VERN"

50 PULL-UPS
RUN 400 METERS
100 PUSH-UPS
RUN 400 METERS
150 SIT-UPS
RUN 400 METERS
200 AIR SQUATS
RUN 400 METERS
250 DOUBLE UNDERS

STRENGTH

Don't focus on flying through this one! Focus on form and function. Get in tune with your body and dial in on the muscle groups being used. Pay attention to how the body works together as a WHOLE! If this is too easy… add reps. If it's too hard… adjust accordingly. It's all about progression. One day at a time!

Complete 10-15 reps and 3 rounds of the following…

1. PUSH-UPS
2. LEG RAISES
3. AIR SQUATS
4. SIT-UPS
5. HAND RELEASE PUSH-UPS
6. REVERSE LUNGE
7. CRUNCHES
8. CHAIR/BENCH DIPS

ADVANCED WOD
"THE SEVEN"
SEVEN ROUNDS OF THE FOLLOWING:
7 HSPU'S (HANDSTAND PUSH-UPS)
7 THRUSTERS 135/95
7 KNEES TO ELBOWS
7 DEADLIFTS 245/165
7 BURPEES
7 KB SWINGS 70/53
7 PULL-UPS

HIT

Set your timer for 30 seconds of work, 15 seconds of rest, 6 cycles. Perform each of the following movements at 100% effort for 30 seconds followed by a short 15 second break. During the 15 seconds of rest gear up for the next movement on the list! Complete 30 seconds of each and then rest 90 seconds between rounds. **Total time:** 24:30 - 29:00

Warm-up
5 minutes of brisk walking, jogging in place, jumping rope, etc.

Complete HIIT Cycle 3-4X
1. JUMP ROPE
2. BEAR CRAWLS
3. JUMPING LUNGES
4. BUTT KICKERS
5. JUMP TUCKS
6. PLANK

OPTIONAL CASHOUT:
100 DOUBLE UNDERS
-OR- 300 JUMP ROPES

ADVANCED WOD
"THE 100"
100 DOUBLE UNDERS
90 PUSH-UPS
80 SIT-UPS
70 AIR SQUATS
60 PULL-UPS
50 DIPS
40 BOX JUMPS 24/20
30 BURPEES
20 TOES TO BAR
10 HSPU'S

STRENGTH

Did you know that BUILDING MUSCLE is the quickest and most efficient way to burn fat? Fact. Time to sculpt those arms and legs! Complete the rep count for each bodyweight movement. Remember, this is a slower day so focus on form. Get in tune with those muscles of yours. If you feel like you have more in the tank after 2 rounds… add a 3rd or 4th round, do additional reps of each or add some weight. Get strong!

Warm-up
5 minutes of brisk walking, jogging in place, jumping rope, etc.

20 - SIT-UPS
15 - AIR SQUATS
10 - WALKING PUSH-UPS
5 - PIKED SHOULDER PRESSES
10 - COMMANDOS
15 - SUMO SQUATS
20 - SINGLE-LEG V-UPS
REPEAT 2 - 4x

ADVANCED WOD
"PUSH & PULL"
4 ROUNDS OF THE FOLLOWING:
RUN 400 METERS
10 TRX ATOMIC PUSH-UPS
10 PULL-UPS
10 KB PUSH-UPS
10 TRX LOW ROWS
10 PIKED PUSH-UPS
10 KB BENT ROWS 53/35 R/L
10 KB SWINGS 53/35

SPRINTS

Find a track, park or not-so-busy street and complete this sprint sequence 3 times through. Sprints are a great way to boost your metabolism (along with all the other workouts you've done this week!). High intensity interval training has been proven to be one of the most effective fat burning methods. There are so many different ways to mix it up! Fitness is supposed to be fun! And as you can see from this week of workouts you don't need a lot of time or expensive equipment... all you need is YOU! **Total time:** 22:00

Warm-up

5 minutes of brisk walking, jogging in place, jumping rope, etc.

10 SEC SPRINT/ 10 SEC REST
20 SEC SPRINT/ 20 SEC REST
30 SEC SPRINT/ 30 SEC REST
60 SEC SPRINT/ 60 SEC REST
REST 90-120 SECONDS
REPEAT 3x

ADVANCED WOD
"STADIUM OF FIRE"
4 COMPLETE LAPS
4 STATIONS AROUND THE TRACK
EVERY 100 METERS
STATION 1: 25 BURPEES
STATION 2: 25 KETTLEBELL SWINGS 53/35
STATION 3: 25 MOUNTAIN CLIMBERS
STATION 4: 25 JUMP SQUATS

THE ULTIMATE CLEAN SIMPLE EATS SWAPS AND SUBSTITUTIONS LIST

If you have dietary restrictions or food allergies, you can still use our Clean Simple Eats Meal Plans with these swaps! If you can't find these swaps in store, check online. Amazon and Thrive Market have great options. Keep in mind when making ingredient swaps, the macros for the recipe will change. If you'd like to track your macros accurately, we recommend inputting each recipe into our CSE+ app with individual ingredients.

GENERAL SWAPS:

Avocado: for savory entrees: nuts, cheese, seeds. For sweet recipes such as shakes: canned, full-fat coconut milk, unsweetened coconut flakes or nut butter

Banana: other fruit of choice // example: 50g banana = 140g strawberries, 170g raspberries, 80g blueberries, 80g apples, 115g peaches, 85g pineapple, 75g pears

Bison: lean ground beef

Eggs: for baking: Bob's Red Mill Egg Replacer or replace one egg with 3 Tbs. water + 1 Tbs. ground flaxseed or 3 Tbs. water + 1 Tbs. ground chia seeds or ¼ cup unsweetened applesauce or ½ of a mashed avocado or ½ of a mashed banana or ¼ cup coconut yogurt. For savory breakfast dishes or entrees (use where applicable): diced chicken, deli turkey, turkey bacon or Follow Your Heart brand Vegan Egg

Ezekiel Bread: Dave's Killer Bread Thin Sliced, Harper's Bran Bread, or any 80 calorie per slice whole grain bread

Fish: chicken breast

Ground Turkey: lean ground chicken or lean ground beef

Honey: pure maple syrup

Oats: cream of wheat, farro

Salmon: cod, halibut, mahi mahi or chicken breast

DAIRY:

Butter: coconut oil

Bolthouse Dressing: Daiya dressings, Primal Kitchen or Tessemae's (use half the amount in all brands)

Cheddar Cheese: Daiya brand or Follow Your Heart brand dairy-free cheddar

Chocolate Chips: Enjoy Life or Nestle Simply Delicious chocolate chips

Cottage Cheese: dairy-free yogurt (see Greek yogurt)

Cream Cheese: Daiya brand dairy-free cream cheese

CSE Pancake & Waffle Mix: Annie's Pancake & Waffle Mix, Enjoy Life Pancake & Waffle Mix, or Birch Benders

Feta: Treeline brand cashew cheese

Greek Yogurt: Daiya brand, Silk brand or Kite Hill brand dairy-free plain yogurt

Kodiak Cakes: Annie's Pancake & Waffle Mix, Enjoy Life Pancake & Waffle Mix, or Birch Benders

Laughing Cow Cheese: Daiya brand dairy-free cream cheese or Treeline brand dairy-free soft cheeses

Mayo: Primal Kitchen Mayo, Hellman's Vegan Mayo, Just Mayo, Thrive Market Coconut Oil Mayo, Kraft Olive or Avocado Oil Mayo or make at home

Milk: unsweetened almond milk or cashew milk

Mexican Shredded Cheese: Daiya brand or Follow Your Heart brand dairy-free cheddar

Mozzarella Cheese: Daiya brand dairy-free mozzarella

Parmesan Cheese: Follow Your Heart brand dairy-free shredded Parmesan style cheese

Pepper Jack Cheese: Daiya brand or Follow Your Heart brand dairy-free pepper jack style cheese

Pesto: Vegan, dairy-free basil pesto or make at home

Protein Powder: CSE Vegan Protein Powder (CSE powders are third party tested lactose free)

Ricotta Cheese: Kite Hill dairy-free ricotta

NUTS:

Almond butter: any other nut butter, sunbutter or coconut butter

Almonds: any other nuts

Almond extract: vanilla extract

Almond Milk: cashew milk, coconut milk, hemp milk or skim milk

Cashew Sour Cream: plain Greek yogurt

Cashews: any other nut or seed

Coconut: sunflower seeds, any other nut, any other nut butter, sunbutter

Coconut extract: vanilla extract

Coconut Milk (canned): heavy cream for full-fat, Half and Half for light

Kodiak Cakes: Annie's Pancake & Waffle Mix, Enjoy Life Pancake & Waffle Mix, or Birch Benders

Peanuts: any other nut or seed

Peanut Butter: any other nut butter, sunbutter or coconut butter

Tree-nuts: sunflower seeds, pumpkin seeds, sunbutter, peanuts, peanut butter, coconut, coconut butter

*in savory dishes, any healthy fat may be swapped in for the nuts, i.e. avocado, cheeses, seeds, olives

GLUTEN:

Breadcrumbs: gluten-free breadcrumbs

Buns/Bread: gluten-free bread/buns

CSE Pancake & Waffle Mix: gluten-free Kodiak Cakes Mix, FlapJacked Mix or any other gluten-free pancake mix

Kodiak Cakes Mix: gluten-free Kodiak Cakes Mix, FlapJacked Mix or any other gluten-free pancake mix

Oats: gluten-free rolled oats

Pasta: brown rice pasta

Tortillas: corn or brown rice tortillas

Whole Wheat Flour: All-Purpose gluten-free flour

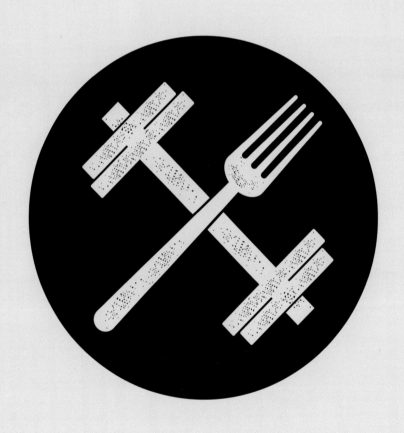

WWW.CLEANSIMPLEEATS.COM